The Art of Lactation

The Loving Milk Maid's
Complete Guide to Making Milk
for the Adult Nursing Couple

Jennifer Elisabeth Maiden

Visit the author's website:
http://www.bountifulfruits.com

For Mr. S with love
Always and Forever...

"A bundle of myrrh is my wellbeloved unto me;
he shall lie all night betwixt my breasts."
Song of Solomon 1:13

FOREWORD

When I stop to consider the events that have transpired in my life, it sometimes feels that I was born a milk maid. My personal journey into the land of lactation, where breast milk flows as sweetly as liquid gold, began well over 14 years ago, following the birth of my first child, when, quite by chance, my husband, known affectionately as Mr. S, and I stumbled upon the beautifully mystifying world of the adult nursing relationship, an exquisite experience that I now share with others through my website, Bountiful Fruits, where I advocate and educate others on this unique--and quite private--lifestyle choice as "The Loving Milk Maid", or simply "LMM".

Over the years, as I have joyfully nursed three healthy and happy children--and one extremely content husband--I have learned a great deal about the art of lactation, and hope to share my knowledge with others who dream of sharing the beloved gift of breast milk with their loving partner.

While the process of making breast milk is a truly magical one, I am afraid that you will find no magic within the pages of this book; rather, you'll discover tried and true methods to naturally--and safely--produce breast milk while building a stronger relationship with your partner. Although I had the privilege of working closely with a small team of registered nurses, board certified lactation consultants, and a certified herbalist during the writing of this book, I am not a qualified medical professional, of course, so it is always advised to discuss specific issues with your health care provider, or a certified lactation consultant.

I warmly embrace my role as a friend and confidante to other nursing couples who seek a kinship with someone who understands the joy and great personal pleasure gained from this most intimate of human experiences. Guiding others along the less-traversed paths of adult nursing and lactation has been a blessing in my life, and having the opportunity to write this book to help you on your own journey into lactation is a true privilege.

With affection,

Jennifer Elisabeth Maiden

LMM

"Let thy fountain be blessed and rejoice with the wife of thy youth. Let her be as the loving hind and pleasant roe; let her breasts satisfy thee at all times; and be thou ravished always with her love."

Proverbs 5:18-19

Part One

Lessons in Lactation

Chapter 1

What is Lactation?

In the very basic definition of the word, lactation can be defined as the formation of breast milk, but when it comes to making that beautiful breast milk, many couples discover that the process can be a true labor of love, one that takes a great deal of time, patience, and concentrated effort. Breast milk does not just happen. It must be produced over a sometimes lengthy period of time, and if you are hoping to accomplish the goal of making breast milk without the aid of pregnancy and/or childbirth, which, of course, makes the process much easier, then you and your partner will need to take a very realistic approach to lactation. Producing breast milk requires a great deal of physical and emotional responsibility, and just like the beautiful nursing relationship itself, lactation is a partnership where you will work together to build--and maintain--a healthy supply of breast milk.

The process of producing non-maternal breast milk is referred to as inducing lactation or lactation induction, and it is a very real and exciting possibility for every woman. Over the years, many women have successfully induced lactation and enjoyed a healthy supply of breast milk, even if they have never experienced pregnancy or childbirth, are post-menopausal, or have undergone hysterectomies. The process requires a perfectly balanced cocktail of hormones such as progesterone, prolactin, estrogen, and oxytocin, which are released by the pituitary gland, located at the base of the brain, which means that very little can hinder a woman's ability to make breast milk.

When a woman has previously lactated and chooses to induce lactation at a later period in her life, this process is called re-lactation. In essence, the re-lactating woman is reminding her body of what it has previously done, and this can sometimes speed up the milk-making process.

Lactation can be an emotionally stressful and physically taxing process for the woman, particularly if she feels that she isn't producing milk quickly enough, or in the desired amount. It's extremely important that she remains relaxed and focused, as stress can inhibit breast milk production and flow, and that her partner remains supportive and encouraging during this period in her life. Lactation is a journey, sometimes a lengthy one full of twists and turns, but it's a beautiful part of the nursing experience, as the process of working together to induce lactation builds intimacy and helps to create an unbreakable bond between two loving people. The induction process is something to be enjoyed and celebrated every step of the way. Once you reach your final destination, you'll understand the value of that long and arduous trip.

Lactation can be gauged by two levels: partial lactation, in which the nursing couple enjoy producing and sharing some breast milk while retaining a great deal of flexibility within their busy lifestyle, and full lactation, in which there is a greater volume of milk, but less convenience. Many couples find that partial lactation is a beautiful option as they strive to create a healthy balance between the hectic chaos of everyday life and their nursing relationship. The beautiful thing about lactation is the choice it provides to the loving nursing couple. If you reach partial lactation and choose to later pursue full lactation, you can do so by increasing the number of suckling sessions you share, and incorporate pumping sessions into your daily induction routine. If you someday realize that full lactation is not as enjoyable, or far more challenging, than you had expected it to be, you can return to a stage of partial lactation by eliminating additional pumping sessions and reducing the number of times you nurse per day.

Set a personal lactation goal and commit to it, but don't focus so strenuously on making milk that you lose sight of love and intimacy. Relax and enjoy every moment of this exquisite experience. The beginning of a loving journey into lactation is a new adventure that you and your partner will never have the opportunity to experience again, so be sure to admire the beautiful sights along the way.

Chapter 2

Anatomy of a Woman

Before we explore techniques to induce lactation, and how to draw that lovely milk from the gracious and giving breasts once it has begun to flow, let's take a moment to discus the beautiful female breast, how it produces milk, and put to rest two common myths regarding breastfeeding.

The female breast, comprised of specialized glandular tissue and fat cells, overlays the pectoral muscles, and, outwardly is made up of the body, the nipple, and the areola, the ring of color surrounding the human nipple. Housed within these magnificently unique woman's breasts, which have been preparing to produce milk since she was an embryo in her mother's womb, is an intricate network of channels that all work together to produce breast milk. Nestled within each breast are the milk ducts; during the inducing process, a woman will release high levels of progesterone, estrogen, and prolactin, three important hormones that encourage breast milk production. When these hormones are released, the milk ducts increase in number and size.

The ducts branch off into ductulets, which are located near the breast wall, and at the end of each ductulet is a cluster of tiny grape-like sacs called alveoli (plural: alveolus), and these contain milk-producing cells known as lactocytes. A cluster of alveoli is called a lobule, and a cluster of lobules is called a lobe. Each breast contains between 15 and 20 well-organized lobes, with one milk duct for every lobe.

When prompted by prolactin, alveoli take proteins, sugars, and fat from a woman's blood supply to make breast milk. Cells surrounding the alveoli squeeze the glands, pushing the milk into the ductulets, which lead to a bigger duct. Some of these ducts will merge so that approximately eight of them end at the tip of the nipple to deliver milk to the recipient.

There are two common misconceptions when it comes to nursing.

The first states that successful lactation is determined by breast size, and this is inaccurate, as the amount of milk a woman produces is never determined by the size or shape of her breasts. While it is true that larger breasts have the capacity to contain more milk than their smaller counterparts, there is no truth to the myth that they produce more milk.

Another common mistake made by the new-to-nursing couple is thinking that breast milk is stored in the nipple. It is not. The nipple, which contain between four and 20 individual openings, is merely used as a receptacle so that milk can easily flow from the breast. This is why utilizing a proper latch while suckling, which we will explore later, is crucial to successful milk production and flow.

It is very common to experience breast changes during the process of lactation, as volumes of water and electrolytes fill the wall of the breast and cause the skin to stretch in preparation of milk production. Many women's breasts increase 1-2 bra cup sizes during lactation, and a total breast weight gain of 3/4 to 2 pounds may be expected. Due to a surge in blood flow, the areolae often darken and increase in circumference while the nipples enlarge, normally widening at the base, and become erect and protuberant during stimulation. As the skin of the breasts stretch, it often becomes translucent, and veins and blood vessels are more prominent just beneath the surface. These changes can cause a slight shift to the shape of the breast, and this is a perfectly normal part of the lactation process.

The areolae contain small harmless sebaceous glands of Montgomery (or Montgomery glands), which become much more prominent during lactation. These glands are rich in very good, natural oils that protect and lubricate the nipple while releasing an enzyme that kills bacteria during nursing.

It is also common to experience a feeling of heaviness, or a slight tingling or prickling sensation as your breasts undergo this incredible new change. Tenderness in the underarm area and tender places in the breast, particularly along the outer side, are also normal, and you may even experience small shooting "growing pains" as the process of lactation continues.

This is a time for celebration as your breasts metamorphose into beautiful new nursing breasts.

Not only is every woman's breast unique, but every breast is, too, and you may experience different changes in each of your own breasts. The fear of stretch marks and ptosis, the medical term for sagging, often arises, but how much your breasts change depends a great deal on heredity and genetics.

Always remember, nursing breasts are a beautiful sign of womanhood and femininity. Treasure them, and do not forget that a man who appreciates the beauty of these breasts is one who appreciates the essence of a woman.

Chapter 3

Categories of Milk

As your body begins the beautiful process of lactation and starts to produce nature's finest food, that nutrient-enriched liquid gold, you will notice a difference in the type of milk your body makes.

In the beginning, the breasts produce colostrum, sometimes referred to as first milk. Thick and yellow in color, colostrum is rich in protein, antibodies, vitamins, and minerals.

Your body will then begin to produce transitional milk, which replaces colostrum. Transitional milk is thin and white and contains high quantities of fat, calories, protein, lactose, and vitamins.

Finally, transitional milk will be replaced by the production of mature milk. Mature milk consists mostly of water, and will appear bluish in color when first expressed. This is called foremilk. As milk continues to flow and its fat content increases, it transforms into white hindmilk. Hindmilk is very important if milk is being consumed for its health properties, as it is packed with nutrients.

There is no such thing as weak or bad breast milk. Even though the consistency and flavor, from tangy to sugary-sweet, varies among these milks, they are all very good for you, and perfectly safe to drink, so enjoy!

How soon you will begin to produce any of these milks is dependent upon your body, and how quickly it transitions into a state of lactation. Remember, breast milk changes from day to day, too, so if you see a noticeable difference in the color or consistency, or even the amount you are producing, don't worry! This is just another part of the beautiful journey into lactation!

Chapter 4

Understanding the Supply and Demand
of Lactation

Since you and your partner have chosen to introduce lactation into your loving ANR, you can probably imagine how thrilling it is when those first glistening drops of breast milk appear after all of the hard work you've gone through to make it happen! It's empowering! Emotions run high. You'll be excited and elated, and unable to believe that your body was able to do something so amazing, as your partner anticipates that first sweet taste.

There won't be much at first. But do not be disappointed.

As wonderful as it would be to achieve full milk supply right away, the reality is that lactation takes time, it can be a slow (sometimes frustrating) process, and it varies greatly and is unique to every woman because we are unique--and so are our bodies.

It's sort of cute to think of having our own little milk factories tucked inside our bodies, isn't it? We can make as much fresh, healthy milk as we like--just not in great quantities right away. We "natural milk maids", unfortunately, cannot immediately fill massive orders for the goods. We work on a supply and demand basis.

If you and your partner have dreamed of suckling full, milky breasts just after one nursing, but have only managed to produce a drop or two after several nursing sessions, don't be discouraged. By following a strict set of lactation techniques, and with diligent effort, and a lot of determination, you'll reach the level of lactation you desire.

As you continue your nursing sessions and

produce a little more milk with each feeding, you may find that as your partner suckles he seems to be receiving less milk per feeding, particularly if he is nursing more than once a day. Trust me, he isn't. He is actually emptying your breasts, which is a good thing, as it will aid in a higher level of lactation.

But you want more milk right away, and it seems that it builds up if you allow him to nurse less frequently.

Uh-oh. You've fallen into the milk hoarding trap!

It isn't a good idea to allow milk to build up in the breasts just so your partner will have larger quantities during feedings. This is extremely counterproductive, as it tells your body that you have enough breast milk and it doesn't need to make any more. Remember, supply and demand. The more often your "customer" returns, the more product you will need to produce. If no one is coming by to sample the goods, then there is no reason to make more.

If your goal is to fully lactate, then it is best to empty those breasts, whether by nursing (best choice), manual expression, or pumping. (And once it is empty, stay on the breast for an additional five minutes more if possible to encourage production.) Those empty breasts send a signal to all of those important hormones (like estrogen, prolactin, and oxytocin) inside of you that encourages them to make more breast milk.

The lactation process, sometimes referred to as milk synthesis, is comprised of three stages: Lactogenesis I, II, and III. During breast milk production, the first two phases of Lactogenesis rely heavily on proper placement of hormones, but by the time you have established full lactation, entering Lactogenesis III, hormones play a lesser role in milk synthesis, and milk removal becomes key.

Hence, the supply and demand of lactation.

Breast milk contains a small whey protein known as Feedback Inhibitor of Lactation (FIL). FIL slows milk synthesis when the breast is full. When milk accumulates in the breast, more FIL is present, which causes the production process to slow down. Synthesis then speeds up when the breast is empty, and less FIL is present.

The hormone prolactin must be present for milk synthesis to take place. On the walls of the lactocytes (the milk-producing cells of the alveoli) are prolactin receptor sites, and these allow prolactin in the blood stream to move into the lactocytes and stimulate the synthesis of breast milk. When the alveolus is full of milk, the walls expand, stretch, and alter the shape of the prolactin receptors, which means the hormone cannot enter those sites, which causes a decrease in breast milk. When milk is emptied from the alveolus, the prolactin receptors return to their normal shape, and then allow prolactin to pass through, which, of course, increases breast milk supply. In the very early weeks of full lactation, frequent milk removal increases the number of receptor sites in the breast. More sites mean more prolactin, and that means more breast milk!

When we combine these factors, what do we now know?

Full breasts equal slower milk production, and empty breasts equal faster milk production.

Always remember, a loving ANR is not about milk; it is about intimacy and the desire to share a comforting closeness with your partner. Sometimes, we begin to focus so much attention on one thing that we lose sight of what's truly meaningful. Continue to work on your lactation level, but concentrate on the bond you are creating with your partner.

However, if milk flow is a primary goal in

your own personal ANR journey, then remember that some milk is better than no milk, and it is much more than you had before you began.

Now, go empty your breasts--and don't hoard the milk!

Chapter 5

Coping with Breast Milk Fluctuation

It is always so exciting to see--and taste--those first drops of breast milk, but what happens when the flow unexpectedly stops? It can be disappointing, frustrating, and discouraging, but it is jut another part of the journey into lactation, and it isn't uncommon.

Inducing lactation to produce breast milk is sometimes a slow process that takes a great deal of time and patience to accomplish, particularly if you have never lactated before, and along the way, some women experience a noticeable fluctuation in their milk supply. This is very common, especially   in the beginning. During the lactation process, a woman's brain, body, and breasts perform a fine balancing act; some hormone levels drop while others rise so the breasts will begin to produce milk. Unfortunately, it can take some time to establish a comfortable routine, but over time, as your body adapts to these new changes, it will begin to respond much faster to your signals. Try not to be discouraged--even new mothers who have the benefit of natural lactation on their side can find that it takes weeks--or even months--to establish the perfect nursing routine.

You may have noticed that, in the very beginning of the induction process, you are making a few drops of colostrum--and that your partner can taste it while nursing. This is a wonderful sign that your body is responding to your signals! Believe it or not, the cease of that fabulous colostrum is actually a wonderful thing because it is giving way to proper milk. Isn't that exciting? Nature is simply taking her beautiful course. The milk is there. It is slowly building. Your breasts just aren't quite ready to release it. But they will...in time. There is really nothing you can do to make the process move along more quickly, but you can coax it in the right direction!

Here are some tips to ensure that your personal lactation journey moves along as smoothly as possible:

Always stay relaxed. Stress (including the fear that you are no longer producing milk) impedes lactation. It is important that you remain relaxed and calm and emotionally attuned to the experience. Try not to be a "biological clock watcher". Every woman is unique, and her body will begin the lactation process when it is right for her. Enjoy every step of the way!

Remember to stay on schedule. This is especially important during the first 30 days of the lactation inducing process. During this time, you are "training" your body to make milk, and it will begin to respond to its new schedule.

Regularity is key to successful lactation. If you have already established a nursing schedule, you have begun to send "lactation signals" to your body. If you are truly concerned about your fluctuating milk supply, you can nurse right at your set time without taking advantage of flexible time windows. Do your best to nurse on time for 30 consecutive days to establish routine.

During a nursing session, it is often very helpful if your partner feeds alternately from each breast. When we first began to establish lactation, my husband would nurse from the right breast for 5 minutes, and then nurse from the left breast for 5 minutes, alternating until he had nursed a full 20 minutes from each side. Doing this seems to "prime" the breasts and aid in terrific milk flow!

It is really important to ensure that your breasts are completely empty to encourage breast milk production and flow. Empty breasts become full breasts, as milk production is based on supply and demand. If your breasts are not empty, they will automatically assume that there is no need to make more milk. To ensure that your breasts are empty, your partner needs to properly suckle for a minimum of 20 minutes per breast, even if he is not receiving colostrum or proper milk. If you're worried that this isn't an adequate amount of suckling, he can remain on the breast for an additional 10 minutes, but after 30 minutes, suckling becomes ineffective. Your body needs time to replenish its milk supply, and will become unresponsive to suckling after a half an hour. (If you enjoy the feeling, then, by all means, keep him on the breast! Just remember, it won't help to increase the lactation process.) You can incorporate breast compressions to ensure empty breasts, too.

It is perfectly fine to include additional suckling sessions into your daily routine, as they aid in stimulation; just be sure to nurse at your regularly scheduled time, too. Adding is wonderful, subtracting is not.

Building a breast milk supply with the person you love is a beautiful and rewarding part of the nursing relationship! The longer it takes, the more time you will have to be together, the deeper the level of intimacy you'll share, and the stronger bond you'll create. There is no hurry. Your final destination awaits--be sure to take a moment to enjoy the beautiful sights along the way!

Chapter 6

The Let-Down Reflex

A woman's body is an amazing thing, and although it may seem that making milk is a magical process, there are no black-tipped wands or smoke and mirror tricks to aid in increasing the speed of non-maternal lactation.

A common problem among new-to-nursing couples who have chosen to induce lactation within their loving ANRs is often not how much milk is produced during each feeding session, but how long it takes for the breasts to release it, particularly for the male partner (sorry, guys!) who dreams of full, firm, milk-filled breasts and enjoying a mouthful of liquid gold upon initial contact. It's a nice dream, but unfortunately, the milk-making process simply doesn't work that way.

During a nursing session, the breasts must first release the milk that has been made, and allow it to flow, and this process is known as the let-down reflex.

A woman's body and brain must cooperate and work together as a team to ensure proper lactation. If you have explored the second chapter in this book, then you'll recall how the process of lactation takes place; much of it is brought about by breast stimulation and the proper placement of hormones. When the nerve endings in the nipple and areola are stimulated, the brain receives a signal to release prolactin (which tells the alveoli to gather proteins and sugars from the blood and turn them into milk) and oxytocin (which causes the cells surrounding the alveoli to contract and eject milk down the milk ducts). And this all comes together to create the let-down reflex.

The let-down reflex doesn't just happen. It

is a triggered reflex, normally brought about by suckling (and applying the proper latch technique during nursing sessions). If a woman's partner does not think he is receiving an adequate amount of breast milk quickly enough, he may suck faster and harder to aid in drawing the milk out, and this is counterproductive to the flow of breast milk. Slow, steady, rhythmic suckling is necessary to stimulate the breast and encourage milk production. The let-down reflex can happen within seconds--or may take several minutes. Dedicated nursing takes a lot of patience and practice.

A poor or slow let-down reflex can be caused by many emotional factors such as anxiety, fear, embarrassment, anger, resentment, irritation, or frustration, and can also be attributed to fatigue, poor suckling, stress, and even negative remarks.

This is why support and open lines of

communication are vital to a successful ANR (and the reason that knowledge really is power!). If a woman is feeling the pressure to produce, or is worried that she isn't pleasing her partner, she is going to become tense--and she is not going to be able to make and release milk. Frustration and the sense of failing can cause couples to completely abandon the idea of incorporating a beautiful ANR into their foundation relationship. But you should always remember that you can fully enjoy an adult nursing relationship without seeing a single drop of milk.

"But milk is our main goal. I think I can feel it in there, but it just won't come out!"

All right then. Let's talk more about the let-down reflex, and what you and your partner can do to improve the process and ensure a more pleasant nursing session.

The let-down reflex can actually happen many times during a feeding, and here are some common signs to look for if you're curious as to whether or not your body is working its magic:

- Tingling or fullness in the breasts
- Leakage from the opposite breast
- Uterine contractions
- A sense of calm relaxation or peace
- Drowsiness
- Thirst
- A change in your partner's suckling (from short, rapid "pacifier sucks" to a slower, steadier rhythm)

Not every woman responds the same way, of course, and as time goes by, and you and your partner become accustomed to nursing, these "let-down signs" will become less obvious (and you may not experience them at all). You might not even realize that your body is "letting down"--but it probably is!

There are several tried and true let-down reflex cues that you can try prior to nursing sessions. I have had great success with them, as they help tremendously in the feeding process! I have employed these cues while breastfeeding three children (and one really content husband), and recommend them to nursing wives and breastfeeding mothers. For these cues to be completely effective, you have to relax and use either one--or several in combination-- before you put your partner to the breast and while he is there.

Begin by taking several long, deep relaxing breaths to ease and release tension, and start to visualize by closing your eyes and envisioning your partner at the breast as you use your mind to listen to the sound of his voice. Breathe in the scent of his pillow, or a piece of clothing that he has recently worn. Visualization actually focuses on much more than sight. It is a method of using all the senses to paint a complete picture.

Get comfortable and drink a glass of water or a cup of tea. Avoid any unnecessary distractions, and consider listen to soft music, choose a favorite song that stirs up familiar emotions.

It is helpful to share skin to skin contact by nursing completely naked or nude from the waist up, and include massage by asking your partner to gently rub your shoulders or back, even while he is nursing,

There are methods of preparing your body for let-down, too, and these are a terrific way for your partner to become involved. You can take a warm bath or shower (either alone or together) prior to nursing, gently massage the breasts, roll and/or lightly tug the nipples (or ask him to do this), or apply a warm compress or heating pad to the breasts, shoulders, and back.

An interesting fact is that you can actually

train your body to trigger the let-down reflex, and it's a very simple process.

Our bodies truly do like routines and scheduling. This is why regular and dedicated nursing sessions are so important to successful lactation and milk flow. Unless absolutely necessary, you shouldn't alter or vary your feeding time(s). When your body has come to learn that (as in my case) 11 p.m. is "feeding time", then it will respond accordingly, and may not realize that it is "supposed" to be making milk at 7:00. So, always do your very best to stay on schedule! (It truly does help!)

Create a pre-nursing "trigger routine" for yourself--and stay with it. This can be something as simple as employing a variety of the let-down cues, indulging in your favorite drink, or reading a chapter in a beloved book. Whatever method(s) you decide to use, apply them to your daily nursing routine just before feeding. The soothing feeling of deep breathing, the flavor of your favorite tea, the melody of a special song will trigger your senses and remind your breasts that it's time to make milk. Consistency is key.

And to the loving suckling partner, a true committed and dedicated ANR really is a partnership in every way. It requires support, love, understanding, and a deep emotional connection (as well as a basic understanding of how the female anatomy works). You will be working side by side to ensure that the nursing relationship grows and flourishes. You are responsible for the other's needs and happiness.

Negatively critiquing the nursing woman's ability to quickly produce large quantities of milk is not conducive to a healthy nursing relationship--so don't do it. Causing her to worry that she isn't wholly pleasing you damages a healthy nursing relationship--so don't do it. Love her. Encourage her. Be there for her. Help her. Support her. Hug her. And always stay positive!

Remember, it may be her job to make that lovely milk, but it is your job to coax it from her giving breasts, and in the next chapter, we will discuss the suckling technique you should use to do so!

Chapter 7

The Proper Latch

We are born with the instinct to suckle. From the moment we emerge from our mother's womb, it is in our nature to seek her breast, but over time, as we mature and develop and nature takes her sweet course, we lose the ability to properly latch and suckle, as we are meant to find our sustenance by other means. Fortunately, for those of us who enjoy healthy adult nursing relationships, this instinct can be re-learned fairly easily.

Breast play, where the nipple is licked, sucked, and lavished with the lips and tongue as a form of sexual gratification is a fantastic part of a healthy relationship, but it does not provide the stimulation required to produce breast milk. In an adult nursing relationship, we suckle, even if we dry nurse without the goal of lactation.

Surprisingly, the nipple plays a very small role in suckling. Suckling is oral massage of the areola. Remember that the nipple is merely a very pretty little receptacle that allows milk to pass from the breast into the mouth. When suckling, you should stay off the nipple, especially if you hope to encourage lactation.

Before the proper latch can occur, the breast must be positioned correctly. Many new to nursing women make the mistake of offering the breast by grasping it and pulling back, in an effort to further extend the nipple. To properly offer the breast to her partner, the woman should hold it in a cradled C-shape with one hand, which allows the nipple to remain flat against the areola. This sometimes alters the breast into something of a cone-shape, which makes the latch much easier. It is also quite easy to latch if the woman's breast falls naturally into her partner's mouth.

Here are step-by-step instructions to help you master the art of suckling:

1. Before suckling, find a nursing position that is comfortable for both of you.

2. The nursing partner's mouth needs to be open very wide to ensure that he is taking in as much of the breast as he comfortably can. The lips will be slightly flanged, which means the upper lip will bow upward slightly, and the bottom lip will bow downward. This creates a seal around the areola.

3. The breast must be positioned correctly in the mouth. Think of this placement as a "center-and-aim" position. Center the breast in the mouth and aim toward the back of the throat. The tip of the nipple will be very far into the mouth when using the motion.

4. The tongue then rolls backward in a

smooth motion, and catches the base of the nipple where it connects to the areola. This motion also catches the areola. The tongue is then used to pull the nipple onto the roof of the mouth where it is held in place with firm, but gentle pressure. During suckling, the tongue actually squeezes the base of the nipple, pressing it upward, which coaxes milk to flow from the breast.

5. Draw inward, using your lips to pull the breast into your mouth. Suckling requires control of the mouth rather than the muscles of the jaw, which often eases nursing fatigue and pain. This inward draw allows your tongue to naturally massage the base of the nipple while the lips stimulate the areola in an up and down motion. You can increase your suction simply by using more force when pulling your lips inward. Think of this as pulling your lips against your teeth; it's the same motion.

6. The seal created around the areola

should be tight, but never painful. A woman can check this seal by paying close attention to her partner's lips, or by sliding the tip of a finger against the corner of his mouth. If there is a noticeable gap that allows the fingertip to slide into the mouth with little resistance, then the seal is too loose, and her partner should increase suction. If there is no gap between the corner of the mouth and the breast, then he is latched properly, and can begin to suckle!

7. It is really helpful if the woman is relaxed during the nursing experience, as this allows her breast to remain relaxed and receptive to suckling. Suckling can be described as a gentle pumping motion that pulls the breast forward. When properly suckled, the breast will flatten, which allows for fantastic stimulation while also aiding in the process of lactation.

Suckling occurs in two phases. Both should be smooth and rhythmic, as harsh and forceful sucking is both ineffective and sometimes harmful. Harsh sucking can cause milk ducts to collapse, impeding milk production and flow, and even cause injury to the breast. Be gentle. Nursing should never be painful!

The first suckling phase is used to aid in the let-down reflex, and is a rapid succession of lip movements that pulls quickly against the breast. The second phase is used to receive milk that has begun to flow from the breast. The mouth slows its motion, pacing the inward draw in the classic "suck-swallow rhythm".

If it seems that suckling requires a great deal of coordination, don't worry! It's much easier than you think; it often comes back as second nature once you know how it's done. It might take a bit of practice to master the technique, but part of the fun of nursing is learning how--and learning together.

Chapter 8

Proper Breast Support

Also called the palmer grasp, the C Hold is used to support the breast as you are latching your partner prior to nursing. Breast support gives you the ability to control the movement of your breast and easily guide the nipple into your partner's mouth. It can be used in either the traditional "bulls-eye" or asymmetrical latch.

To use the C Hold support, place your breast in the palm of your hand with your thumb on top, and your fingers curled underneath it. In this hold, your hand will literally form the shape of a letter C. Once your breast is supported, you can squeeze your fingers and thumb together to flatten the areola, which often makes latching much easier. Be sure to keep your thumb and fingers behind the areola and out of the way of your partner's mouth so the latch is not broken and suckling is not disrupted.

The C Hold is especially helpful if a woman has large breasts or small hands. Women with small breasts or larger hands may prefer to use the V Hold method of support.

Also called the scissor grasp, like the C Hold, the V Hold is used to support the breast as you are latching your partner prior to nursing. To use this support effectively, you'll have to be able to spread your fingers very wide to reach far enough behind the areola to be sure that they are not in the way of your partner's mouth, which can break his latch and disrupt suckling.

To use the V Hold support, your areola will be placed between your index and middle finger. Your thumb and index finger will be on top of your breast and your middle, ring, and little finger will be beneath it.

The V Hold is especially helpful if a woman has small breasts or larger hands.

No matter which hold you prefer and find more comfortable, they are each a wonderful way to provide additional breast support, particularly when you and your partner are first learning to nurse. As you grow more accustomed to the suckling experience, you may find, over time, that no breast support is required at all.

Chapter 9

The Bulls-Eye Latch

The traditional bulls-eye technique is one of the oldest methods for latching on, and is commonly taught to new breastfeeding mothers. As its name suggests, the center of the areola and the nipple is the nursing partner's target. This technique works perfectly with the cradle hold. When using the bulls-eye latch, you will hold your breast with your free hand and guide your nipple into your partner's open mouth.

As soon as he has opened his mouth very wide, and you have positioned your nipple slightly upward and towards the center of his mouth, you can quickly pull him in towards you by using the arm that is supporting his head. You want to get as much of the areola into his mouth as possible; he will not be able to aid in the inducing process, or help with proper milk removal, if he is only suckling at the nipple.

When a nursing partner is not properly positioned on the breast, this is known as a shallow latch, which can cause a great deal of nursing discomfort and nipple pain. With a proper latch, the nipple will be very far back into your partner's mouth, and he will use his lips to compress the milk sinuses that lie behind the nipple. His tongue will lie beneath the breast, and over his bottom teeth, and then roll backward, pressing the nipple upward in a squeezing motion that helps to draw milk from the breast.

When using the bulls-eye technique, you can combine it with the proper latch tips provided in Chapter 7 for greater success.

Chapter 10

The Asymmetrical Latch

The asymmetric latch is similar to the more traditional bulls-eye latch, but rather than helping to center your partner to directly latch onto the nipple, you will help him latch slightly off-center. When he uses the asymmetrical latch, he will take in more breast tissue close to his lower jaw and tongue rather than getting some areola tissue above the nipple and some areola tissue below the nipple. By having more tissue contact with his tongue and lower jaw, your baby's tongue and lower jaw, your partner will be able to remove milk from the breasts more easily and effectively.

Just as he will do with any latching technique, your partner will need to open his mouth very wide to properly use the asymmetrical latch. He should aim his mouth just below your nipple, so that his lower lip and chin are lined up just below it. He will connect first with the areola, and after he has taken it into his mouth and begun to suckle, you can help him move his mouth over the nipple so that he has both breast tissue and the nipple in his mouth.

The asymmetrical technique is a fabulous method to use when first starting out, or if your partner has had difficulty with latching or effective suckling to draw milk from the breasts. It works especially well with the cross-cradle hold, and the C hold method of breast support. Some women feel that it's more comfortable than other traditional latches, too.

Just as you would with the traditional bulls-eye latch, be sure to combine this latch with the proper latching techniques you learned in Chapter 7 to ensure nursing success.

Chapter 11

Adult Nursing Positions
for the Loving Couple

There are many nursing positions to choose from, and it is wonderful to try several of them to find the one that works perfectly for both of you to ensure the most pleasant of suckling experiences. Nursing should always be an enjoyable and relaxing experience, so settle in and get comfortable before you begin!

Nursing an adult is wonderful because the close proximity of these loving positions allows you to stroke, caress, and embrace one another during each session, which enhances the intimacy and bond within the relationship. When using these positions, it is often helpful to incorporate pillows or other means of support, and while some positions may not work for every couple, due to breast size, height difference, or pain issues that stem from prior medical conditions, many can be slightly adjusted and customized to you, and your personal preference. Along with providing closeness, many of these positions allow a couple to transition easily into sex either during, or directly after, a nursing session. Experiment with each, and have a lovely time while doing so!

1. The Cradle Hold

The Woman's Position:

In the cradle hold, you will be sitting upright. In a bed, you will need to support your neck, shoulders, and lower back with pillows, and elevate your legs by placing one or more pillows beneath your knees. You will also want to place additional pillows across your lap to help elevate and support your partner.

If nursing from the right breast, you will support your partner's head in the crook of your right arm. Your left hand will provide breast support. When he is nursing from the left breast, your partner's head will be in the crook of your left arm, and you will provide breast support with your right hand.

The Partner's Position:

You will lie on your side, stomach to stomach, with your partner. Your body will either be horizontal or diagonal, and the back of your head will be supported by the bend of her arm. In the cradle hold, your upper body will be supported by pillows and your shoulders and hips will be perfectly aligned.

Quick Tip:

While this position works wonderfully with the bulls-eye latch, larger-breasted women may find this nursing position a bit challenging without the aid of proper (and sometimes additional) breast support.

2. The Cross Cradle Hold

The Woman's Position:

In the cross-cradle hold, you will be sitting

upright. In a bed, you will need to support your neck, shoulders, and lower back with pillows, and elevate your legs by placing one or more pillows beneath your knees. You will also want to place additional pillows across your lap to help elevate and support your partner.

If you're nursing from your right breast, your left arm will cross over your body, and you will use your left hand to bring your partner's mouth to your breast. It may be easier to help him latch if you place your thumb and fingers behind his head, just below his ears. Your right hand will provide breast support. When nursing from your left breast, use your right hand in the same way: arm across your body, hand gripping the back of your partner's head, and allow your left hand to provide breast support.

The Partner's Position:

In this nursing position, you will lie on your side and rotate your body so that your chest and stomach are facing your partner. If nursing from her left breast, position your lower body horizontally or diagonally to the right. Your upper body will be supported by pillows and your shoulders and hips will be perfectly aligned. When switching to the second breast, you will need to rotate your body in the opposite direction.

Quick Tip:

The cross-cradle hold works perfectly with the asymmetrical latch, and is often very helpful when couples are first learning to nurse, or the partner has had trouble latching in the past.

3. Reclining Side by Side

The Woman's Position:

In the reclining side by side position, you will be lying on your side. In a bed, you may want to use pillows to slightly elevate your bottom shoulder and arm. You can either offer your partner your breast using the C or V hold, or allow him to provide breast support.

The Partner's Position:

In this nursing position, you will lie on your side, facing your partner. It may be helpful to use pillows to elevate your hed, bottom shoulder, and arm. Your hands will be free to provide breast support, allowing you to position the breast in your mouth, or to massage your partner's shoulders and back while nursing.

Quick Tip:

This relaxing position provides a great deal of intimacy as two people lie on their sides, facing one another, and gaze into each other's eyes, encourages a great deal of skin to skin contact, and allows the nursing partner to easily support and massage the breast during the suckling experience. It is also wonderful, as hands are free to roam, adding gentle touch to the session. Women with larger breasts may find that they do require additional support when nursing in this position.

4. The Sling Feed

The Woman's Position:

In this nursing position, which is also known as the dangle feed, you will allow your breasts to fall naturally into your partner's mouth, which often prevents the need for breast support while easing any jaw fatigue the partner may experience. In a bed, if your partner is lying down, you will comfortably lean over him, using the mattress, or his shoulders, to support your weight. If sitting upright, use pillows to support your back, neck, and shoulders, and before taking your partner's head into your lap, place additional pillows across your thighs to help elevate his upper body and ease discomfort.

The Partner's Position:

In a reclining position, lie flat on your back, using pillows to support and elevate your head as your partner leans over you and allows her breasts to fall naturally into your mouth. You will need to employ the proper latch even in this position, and your hands will be free to guide her breast into proper suckling position. You will be able to provide sensual breast massage as you suckle. If she is sitting during this position, you will rest your head in her lap with your lower body perpendicular to hers. Rather than stretching upward, which places strain on the neck and jaws, elevate your head, using pillows, to bring yourself up to the level of her breasts.

Quick Tip:

The sling feed is a wonderful way to ensure proper milk removal from the breasts, which encourages production and flow while helping to prevent engorgement, mastitis, blocked milk ducts, and other common nursing maladies. Women with large breasts may find this position very liberating, as it requires no additional breast support, but smaller-breasted women may discover that other positions work better for them.

5. Missionary Supine

In this very intimate position, which allows you and your partner to easily transition from nursing to sex, the woman lies on her back with pillows providing comfortable head, neck, and shoulder support while her partner lies over her to nurse. In this position, it is often easier for the nursing partner to provide adequate breast support. The woman's hands will be free to stroke and caress her partner's face, head, shoulders, or back. If nursing naked, this position provides an amazing amount of intimate skin to skin contact. In a variation of this position, the woman may remain lying flat, or may choose to shift into a semi-sitting position, using pillows to provide back, neck, and shoulder support, as the nursing partner straddles her hips and leans slightly over her to suckle.

6. Kneeling Face to Face

Although this position requires the use of a fairly firm surface to execute, it provides a great deal of intimacy and eye contact, as both partners kneel and face one another during the suckling session. By slightly arching her back, the woman can easily offer her breasts to her partner, and may choose to support them using either the C or V hold. In this position, the nursing partner can provide support to one breast while gently massaging the other as he nurses, and the woman can easily support herself by holding on to his shoulders or cradling the back of his neck.

Quick Tip:

This position is not always ideal if there is a significant height difference between the couple. If they feel comfortable doing so, either partner may use pillows or other means of support, beneath themselves to elevate their bodies. Smaller-breasted women, or women whose breasts are firm and slightly more uplifted, may find this position much more convenient than women with larger breasts do.

7. Woman Superior:

Another loving and intimate position that can be used to transition smoothly into sex is the woman superior. In this position, the nursing partner may either recline flat on his back, or relax in a semi-sitting or sitting position, using pillows to provide comfortable neck, shoulder, and back support, while the woman straddles his lap in forward facing position. Because this position allows the nursing partner to provide support and massage to both breasts as he suckles, this position is enjoyable to all women, regardless of breast size and/or shape.

While these seven positions are the most commonly used while enjoying the adult nursing experience, remember, that, with a few minor alterations, *any* position used in a traditional mother-child breastfeeding relationship can be shared and enjoyed by every loving couple.

Chapter 12

Levels of Lactation

Lactation can be measured in 10 levels, beginning with the inducing or re-lactation process, and ending with full lactation, and these measures can be used as a general guideline to help you gauge your personal progress and success as you and your partner work to establish breast milk supply.

Lactation is much more than the physical process of making breast milk; it is also an extremely emotional one, and women often experience a rush of new feelings as the process of inducing begins and her body's hormone levels shift. You might experience bouts of euphoria or tears; some women feel an overwhelming sense of empowerment as they begin the self-discovery of womanhood and recognize their own femininity. You might even notice the urge to "nest". Some women feel the need for greater physical affection, or notice an increase in sexual desire.

The induction of lactation is a wonderful introduction to intimacy and the bonding process as you and your partner work together physically and emotionally to produce that precious breast milk. Even before you see those first glistening drops, you will feel a connection and a sense of accomplishment as a couple.

And as you begin this lovely journey, your breasts will begin the beautiful transformation into nursing breasts, which we explored in Chapter 2. You might feel an urgency to nurse or express throughout the day, even when your partner isn't available to suckle, and don't be surprised if your body responds to the cries (or even coos) of a baby! This maternal response is a very natural and normal part of a woman's make-up.

If suckling is a new experience for you, it

may cause tender nipples and slight breast discomfort throughout the first two weeks, but you'll soon grow accustomed to these new changes, and find that they become very commonplace and a comfortable part of your day-to-day activities. Some women find that they require a more comfortable or supportive bra while others prefer to go bra-less whenever possible.

You might notice a change in your menstrual cycle; this, too, is dependent upon the woman, but chart any changes that you notice, and take a bit of precaution if you're hoping to avoid pregnancy. Contrary to popular belief, a woman can conceive while nursing.

Prior to suckling, your beautiful, brand-new nursing breasts may feel firm and hard; when they feel soft and pliable after a nursing (or pumping) session, you'll know that you have achieved the first of 10 levels of lactation!

Lactation level 2 is one of the most comfortable places to be during the process of inducing milk production. As your body grows accustomed to the new changes it has undergone and your emotions reach a much more even keel as your hormones level off, you may also see a noticeable improvement in your complexion (clear and radiant) and hair (soft and shiny), and an overall feeling of happiness, tranquility, and relaxation as your body continues to release the powerful combination of oxytocin and prolactin during its mission to make milk. At this very early stage in your lactation journey, the need to nurse (or express in your partner' absence) often stems from an emotional desire rather than a purely physical one, which still ensures a great deal of flexibility as you and your partner work to establish a dedicated nursing schedule that suits your lifestyle. During the onset of the second level of lactation, you will be working to make milk rather than working to draw it from the breast. This is often when couples choose how frequently they will nurse, and if they will work to achieve partial or full lactation.

Once you have reached Level 2 in the journey of lactation, two exciting things often occur:

1. During hand expression, you may notice occasional drops of breast milk, and

2. While nursing, your partner will often feel fluid against his tongue

Initially, these drops may be very thick in consistency and dark yellow in color. This is colostrum, sometimes referred to as first milk, and its flavor is sometimes described as being rich and tangy, or even sour. Colostrum is full of fabulous antibodies, and is perfectly safe for your partner's consumption.

Do not over-express your breasts once colostrum is present, or apply harsh, painful pressure in an attempt to draw more colostrum from the breast. This can cause damage and injury to the milk ducts. It is also important for your partner to remember this. It is very exciting to see and taste those first drops, but harder and more forceful sucking is counterproductive; it will not draw more fluid from the breast. It can actually impede the milk-making process by causing the milk duct to collapse. He needs to remain focused and relaxed, and continue with the slow suckling rhythm, while ensuring that he is properly latched. In his eagerness, if he falls off of the breast and attaches only to the nipple, you'll need to re-latch him properly before proceeding with the nursing session.

Another common mistake that new-to-nursing couples often make is opting to express or pump rather than suckle when the opportunity presents itself. Some couples believe that once breast milk is present, it is more beneficial to hand express rather than nurse because they feel that they will draw more milk from the breast by manual stimulation. This is often due to the visual appeal of actually being able to see that lovely milk, but it is inaccurate. While hand stimulation and pumping are fantastic substitutes to employ when your partner is unavailable to nurse, there is no replacement for a suckling mouth. Suckling ensures that the breasts are properly emptied, which encourages further--and greater--milk production, supply, and flow. If you feel the need to express and your partner is available to nurse, definitely put him to the breast! It is much more productive than using hand stimulation or a pump--and it feels nicer, too!

So, what comes next?

By the time you reach Lactation Level 3, you and your partner have probably established a nursing routine that suits your busy lifestyle. At this point in the journey, there is still room to adjust your schedule, and level 3 provides much of the same comfort and flexibility as you found in level 2. During the third phase of lactation, you will continue to work together to produce breast milk, concentrating your efforts on production rather than flow. There may be very little difference in the amount of fluids your partner is receiving in comparison to those of level 2.

You have probably noticed a change in your relationship, even when you are not nursing. You may experience a beautiful rush of new love, and desire your partner's touch throughout the day. You may long for him when he is away, and eagerly wait for his return. Don't be surprised if your libido increases! It often does, and this is just one of the many benefits of sharing a dedicated adult nursing relationship with your life partner!

You may even discover that you are communicating more as you discuss your suckling schedule, choose comfortable feeding positions, and openly talk about the challenges and joys you've found within your nursing relationship, and this is a wonderful way to build that desired level of intimacy and ensure that your connection to one another remains strong.

During this third phase, you may experience your first increase in breast size. Your nursing breasts will continue to swell with the impending promise of milk, and you may feel little "growing pains" as they prepare to sustain your partner, and they will feel soft and pliable to the touch after each nursing session. At this point, a missed nursing should pose no physical discomfort to the breasts. But this will change as you transition into Lactation Level 4.

The fourth phase of lactation is often considered one of three milestone levels in the journey of lactation. At this point, nursing becomes vital, as the desire to be suckled from shifts from being an emotional longing to a physical need. Your breasts have now grown very accustomed to your nursing schedule, and your body has adjusted to--and welcomed--your daily routine. During this beautiful milestone phase, your body is working strenuously to achieve the goal of partial lactation, so if a nursing session is missed, you may experience physical discomfort. It is extremely important that your partner is available to nurse at the allotted suckling time. Typically, a breast pump isn't very effective at this phase, as you'll be unable to release and express milk on your own. You may no longer see the appearance of colostrum during hand stimulation or expression. Don't worry! The milk is there! It is simply building in quantity and waiting to be released by a suckling mouth, as our bodies have intended since the beginning of time. (Go ahead and use that helpful pump to stimulate your breasts, but don't depend on it to empty them just yet!)

During this phase, the possibility of engorgement presents itself to the experience, and it is painful. Not only does engorgement, which can occur in either one or both breasts, cause a lot of physical discomfort, it can make latching very difficult, as the swelling can cause the nipple to retract and flatten against the areola, further impeding the suckling process. It can be very difficult for a woman to enjoy nursing when she is engorged, but if you can tolerate the discomfort, you should continue to nurse if possible. Suckling is really the best cure for engorgement. Prior to nursing, you can take a warm shower or bath, but try to avoid a lot of heat, as this can cause engorgement to worsen, or employ gentle breast massage, or reverse breast stimulation to move the swelling away from the areola. Nurse from the least painful side first. Engorged breasts are often stubborn breasts, so your partner may have some difficulty in drawing milk from the nipple. Remain relaxed, patient, and focused, and encourage him to continue with a gentle suckling rhythm, as he may be tempted to pull forcefully against the breast in hope of really encouraging the release of that milk. You or your partner can incorporate firm and steady breast compressions while nursing to aid in releasing your milk. After 5-10 minutes of nursing without results, move him to the second breast; he can always return to the first side when he has finished. At this phase, it is perfectly fine to nurse outside of your schedule (although you shouldn't skip your "set" time) if you feel the need to do so.

As challenging as Level 4 may seem, it is actually a beautiful phase of lactation. You will begin to see the fruits of your labor, and at this time, you will come to truly depend upon your partner in a way that you never have before. This is such a loving and generous phase, and knowing that you have someone you can fully rely on to fulfill your emotional and physical needs is a fantastic part of any relationship!

There is a reason the fourth level of lactation is often considered one of three milestones within the lactation journey. It requires an exorbitant amount of commitment and responsibility, particularly for the suckling partner, as the lactating woman, who can find this phase quite taxing, must be able to rely on him in a very physical way.

But why is Lactation Level 4 such a milestone?

Because it is the phase that will carry you into the beautiful place of partial lactation.

And if you have come through this milestone, you are well on your way to full lactation--after a pleasurable (and sometimes leisurely) stop by partial lactation. Congratulations! This is truly something to celebrate!

Lactation Level 5 is a reward you'll gain from the hard, dedicated work you put into the previous phase of your lactation journey, and it's a beautiful place to be! You might discover that you are more relaxed, and fully able to enjoy what your body is doing to accomplish the mission of making breast milk as you grow accustomed to routine suckling and pumping sessions. Normally, engorgement is less of a concern during this phase of lactation, as your milk supply continues to increase, and your breasts are much more receptive to pumping in your partner's absence.

There is often a noticeable change in that beautiful supply of breast milk when you have achieved this level of lactation. During nursing sessions, your partner will begin to occasionally swallow milk while suckling.

You may have noticed a change in your menstrual cycle, and this is not an uncommon occurrence as your body goes through the intricate process of lactation. Following childbirth, nursing stimulates the uterus with strong contractions that help to control postpartum bleeding. These uterine contractions often perform the same "trick" in regard to a woman's monthly cycle. A change in your period, particularly if you've never experienced problems in the past, probably stems from nursing. You may see a change in regularity, flow, or length of your cycle, and find that nursing actually helps to ease the difficulties of PMS or menstrual cramps. During this time, you and your partner may notice a decrease in your milk supply, but don't be discouraged by this! It's just your body's way of storing fluids to ensure that you remain healthy and well-balanced. Continue to nurse and pump on schedule, and your milk supply will resume--and continue to increase!

As you experience this new physical change, be sure to chart it for future comparison. It is really important to keep accurate track of your changing cycle, particularly if either the hope of conception or the prevention of pregnancy are factors in your foundation relationship.

During the fifth level of lactation, you might notice that you have begun to respond to your partner in very new and exciting ways. His scent or the sound of his voice may stir a deep and intense emotional pull that brings about the desire to nurse or pump, even in his absence. This is a beautiful feeling, as it shows the level of intimacy that you have reached as a couple. It is also beneficial to the let-down reflex, which aids in successful suckling and pumping.

You may notice very little difference in Lactation Levels 5 and 6. During your transition into the sixth phase of the journey, your breasts may swell once more and increase one bra cup size, but there may be no noticeable change in the amount of milk your partner is consuming during regular nursing sessions. This is normal, as you and your partner are working together to build your milk supply, even as your body is continuing to work toward the goal of achieving full lactation.

Pumping in your partner's absence remains an excellent means of breast stimulation, but is often not effective in drawing milk from the breasts. If you are not yet able to collect expressed milk, don't be disappointed or discouraged. Remember, lactation is a beautiful labor of love that progresses at its own pace over time. You are making milk! It really is there! Your breasts jut aren't quite willing to release it by means other than suckling. But that day will come, and when it does, you'll have something else to celebrate. And while you're working to increase that milk supply, don't forget to take the time to enjoy each step along the path of this exquisite journey.

During the sixth level of lactation you may discover that pumping in your partner's absence is not a necessity, as physical discomfort is less of a concern, and this is what makes this phase so comfortably carefree. By this point, your body is completely attuned to your nursing schedule. There is a pleasant shift in the nursing experience, and this level is often one of leisurely repose.

This is also a wonderful time for communication, as you and your partner decide if you will continue the pursuit of full lactation. Some couples find that they are extremely comfortable with the experience of partial lactation, as it provides them with an adequate supply of breast milk to enjoy while giving them the flexibility that is not afforded by full lactation. At this stage, if choosing to remain partially lactated, suckling is used for enjoyment, and as a means of maintaining milk supply rather than increasing it. During this stage of lactation, you'll have time to make this decision, and if you later choose to embark further into the journey, it's wonderful to know that full lactation is always a beautiful possibility!

Enjoy this plane! It's a lovely one on which to rest!

Again, this is a time for communication as you and your partner decide if you are comfortable with partial lactation, which provides a bit of carefree flexibility, or if you will continue your journey into full lactation, which takes careful consideration and planning. Partial lactation is actually comprised of four "sub-levels": 5 and 6 (early stages), 7 (mid stage), and 8 (the final stage). In choosing to increase your breast milk supply with the goal of full lactation in mind, you'll encounter the second milestone in the journey of lactation once you've reached the eighth phase of the milk-making process.

You may find that you remain partially lactated for quite some time. Lactation is often a slow progression that requires patience and time, and during this phase in lactation, it is not uncommon to see a shift in your milk supply as your body continues to undertake the arduous task of lactation. Some women find themselves bouncing between levels 5 and 6 as they work strenuously to reach the next phase of their journey, and this can be frustrating and discouraging. To move smoothly and comfortably into the seventh phase, remain relaxed and focused (but don't remain so focused that you forget to enjoy the beautiful bonding experience that you share with your partner), and adhere to your nursing schedule. Do your best to avoid missing allotted nursing times. Regularity is key for successful lactation.

Lactation Level 7 is a lovely and rewarding place to be. So much has transpired since you began the journey into lactation, but the sweet promise of even more beauty awaits. By this point, your body has grown very accustomed to your nursing schedule, and suckling has now become second nature. Clocks are no longer a necessity; you will be able to rely on instinct, and it will tell you when it is time to nurse (or pump in your partner's absence).

As your beautiful nursing breasts continue the process of lactation, your partner will probably notice an increase in your breast milk supply as he is now regularly swallowing that fabulous milk during nursing sessions. Your breasts may begin to feel swollen and heavy once more, and you might experience that familiar tingling sensation in your areolae, or the little "growing pains" in your breasts. A return of very mild discomfort in the underarm area or along the sides of the breasts is not uncommon. The desire for your partner and the need to nurse often intensifies.

A wonderful thing is taking place.

You are preparing to transition into the eighth phase of lactation.

Lactation Level 8 is the second of three monumental milestones along the way of this exquisite journey, both physically and emotionally. It's a crucial time for many nursing women, as this exciting, although challenging, phase is what they will endure to experience the joy and beauty of full lactation. In many way, the eighth level of lactation offers a great deal of knowledge to the lactating woman, as it guides her along the way and assists her in understanding what will take place once she is fully lactated, and, now, your dream of producing a full supply of breast milk to further enhance the nursing experience is balanced on the horizon. You are very close now. Isn't it exciting?

This is a milestone level of celebration for many couples--and one to enjoy, as it truly provides an even stronger plane of intimacy between two loving people, who often notice their connection to one another grow deeper during this time.

During the eighth level of lactation, your breasts may become very firm and swollen between nursing sessions, and just before suckling, you may experience a sensation of pressure or a strong internal "pull" or "tug" against your breasts. This is nature's way of reminding you that it is time to nurse. And at this phase in the lactation journey, you must nurse during your scheduled time(s). If you miss a nursing session, your breasts will leak. The mild discomfort you feel prior to a suckling session and the fear of leaking will be eased during the nursing session as long a your partner properly empties your breasts. He should be able to do this quite easily by suckling for 20 minutes per side. You may feel much more comfortable if you tuck a nursing pad into each bra cup, particularly if you're out and about.

During nursing, your partner may find that while he is still regularly swallowing without a fluctuation in frequency, he is receiving more breast milk during the experience. And you will probably find that your need for him has grown. As you rely on him to draw milk from your breasts and view him as a loving, supportive, and dependable partner, the bond that you created with the opening of a dedicated ANR grows deeper, now connecting you at the heart. This is a beautiful part of the experience.

Pumping often remains ineffective for drawing milk from the breasts, although it can help to stimulate and ease discomfort if your partner is unavailable to nurse off-schedule. It is perfectly fine to do this between allotted suckling times, and is helpful in keeping you comfortable. Typically, women are unable to hand express at this point, and this is why your partner's presence is so important during this phase of lactation.

Engorgement once again presents itself during this time, and because you probably won't be able to properly pump or express, it is really important that your partner empties those breasts. Engorged breasts are painful breasts, and this condition makes nursing very unpleasant. Some women find engorgement so uncomfortable that they're unable to nurse their partner until their condition improves, and this can cause a decrease in milk supply; it can also be emotionally stressful for both of you, so do your best to stay on schedule and nurse for the appropriate amount of time.

Enjoy this milestone level of lactation, knowing that you and your partner are on the brink of sharing something beautifully monumental that only two very special nursing people can understand.

Now that you have come this far into the journey, what can you expect to find waiting for you?

A stronger, firmer foundation relationship, an abundance of intimate love, and two extremely rewarding levels of lactation!

You have accomplished the second milestone in your milk-making mission, and learned the importance of balance and planning, as your beautiful nursing breasts helped you to understand both the significance of scheduled suckling and what you will experience once you reach the third and final lactation milestone. This level also provided you with the new understanding of what your breasts are truly capable of, and what you can do as a woman.

By the time you arrive at Level 9, you may find that your overall emotional mood has improved, and it is not uncommon to feel euphoric, carefree, and relaxed, as your body continue to release that magically powerful combination of oxytocin and prolactin during nursing sessions.

From now on, your breasts will have grown very accustomed to the art of producing breast milk and will no longer show great change. They will continue to swell and firm between nursing sessions, and as long as you are sure to suckle on schedule--or pump when necessary, discomfort and leakage should not be serious concerns. Because you now understand your body and breasts, you will be able to relax and fully enjoy this level of lactation.

Lactation Level 9 is a lovely and exciting place to be. You and your partner have experienced so much as a couple since you began the journey into lactation together, and the joy of reaching full lactation is still to come. This is the perfect time for you and your partner to connect emotionally as you openly discuss your feelings on the experience of what you are sharing, what you have accomplished, and what you hope to further gain from your personal ANR. As your beautiful nursing breasts continue the process of lactation, you may notice an increase in your milk supply, and your partner's suck and swallow reflex pattern may change as he is now continuously swallowing that fabulous milk during nursing sessions. While pumping, you may be able to collect some milk, and in between nursing sessions, you may find that you are expressing very small quantities of breast milk.

A wonderful thing is taking place.

You are preparing to transition into the tenth phase of lactation.

Yes. You have reached full lactation.

Lactation Level 10 is the third and final monumental milestone along the way of this exquisite journey, and it is amazing.

This is a cause for celebrating all that you have accomplished and all that you have achieved as a loving and committed couple. The journey may have been a long and sometimes difficult one, but isn't the destination you've reached perfect?

While he is nursing, your partner may now notice two new changes in your breast milk: an increase in quantity and a shift in the way it flows. Before you reach full lactation, your partner may find that milk rolls from the breasts and into his mouth, whereas, when you are fully lactated, it sprays from the breasts and into his mouth.

And this is precisely what you will notice, too! When you have reached the tenth phase in lactation, you will be able to easily pump, hand express, and spray breast milk. It will be very important to keep up with your nursing sessions, as you will now let-down (or leak) much more noticeably than you did in level 8 if you miss a session. Lactation Level 10 provides some flexibility, though, that is very reassuring to many women, because you will now be able to successfully empty your own breasts by hand expressing or pumping, which means you can avoid embarrassing accidents and wet blouses. Be sure that your breasts are empty before you head out to meet the day to protect your private lifestyle choice, and, to increase your own confidence as a fully lactating woman, you might consider lining each bra cup with a nursing pad.

Engorgement now becomes a very real possibility during this time, but because you can hand express and pump in your partner's absence, you will be able to see to your own needs and prevent painful breasts and discomfort, and that is a wonderful thing!

Breast care is also very important for the fully lactated woman. Although you have now grown accustomed to nursing and should no longer experience suckling discomfort that sometimes arises from the newness of breast stimulation or an improper latch, you may notice that the skin of your breasts appears thin and translucent. This is normal, as your breasts have swollen to contain all of that lovely new breast milk! Unfortunately, this can cause the skin to "break down", which is another way to explain a painful tear in your flesh, normally noticed where the skin is pulled the tautest. A lot of times, this happens under the breast, at the base where it connects to the breast wall. It is really important that you make sure your breasts remain completely dry. After nursing or pumping, you should wash them in warm water, and dry them thoroughly. Coconut oil is a terrific addition to your breast care routine; not only does it naturally aid in increasing breast milk supply, it keeps the skin very soft and pliable. Years ago, when I was a young nursing mother (and wife) who worried about "breaking down", I learned an age-old home remedy secret from my grandmother. Cornstarch. I know, it sounds very old-fashioned, but it works! After washing and drying your breasts, you can dust cornstarch on the underside of them, focusing on the area where they meet the wall of the breast. Cornstarch has magical powers, did you know that? It absorbs any moisture and keeps your breasts cool and refreshed while healing any break down. And it's natural and safe for human consumption, so if you forget to brush it off prior to nursing, it won't harm your partner, unlike other perfumed powders. Always remember to change your nursing pads frequently, too.

You may have read that the "average" lactating woman produces between 25 and 40 ounces of breast milk per day. Those numbers normally refer to the amount of milk an exclusively breastfeeding woman makes, and you probably don't have the luxury of exclusively nursing your partner. Don't judge your personal success by numbers. Your milk supply will continue to naturally increase over time, and you can help this along by nursing or pumping as frequently as possible. Too much breast milk can be just as challenging as "not enough" breast milk, because as your supply increases, you'll need to be certain that you keep ahead of it with frequent expressions. But I'm sure you can do it! After all, watching your breast milk increase is part of the fun in full lactation.

If you have reached this phase of lactation in your own nursing relationship, a goal that you have proudly achieved, congratulations! I share in your happiness, and wish you great joy!

This concludes "Lessons in Lactation". Although the first part of the journey has come to an end, the true adventure has just begun as we explore the methods you and your partner can use to begin the lactation process.

Part II

Methods of Making Milk

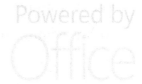

Chapter 1

The Flexible 30-Day Nursing Schedule

A common problem that many active nursing couples who hope to induce lactation within their loving ANR face is finding a nursing schedule that they can commit to. This simple schedule is wonderful because it revolves around your busy lifestyle, and can be completely customized. What's even better is that it will produce results within 30 days with just one dedicated daily nursing session, and without the need of incorporating herbal supplements or additional pumping sessions.

The key to successful lactation is regularity. For this nursing schedule to work, you really need to make time to connect with your partner. There is no better way to induce lactation than with a willing, suckling mouth! Your body will respond beautifully to this schedule, and your breasts will soon understand that the time to make milk has arrived. While your partner is doing his job by stimulating the breast with proper suckling, your body will begin doing her job by producing breast milk,

To begin using this schedule, you should first choose a time that works perfectly for you and your partner. Plan this carefully, as this will become your "set time", the time that your body will adjust to as a means of producing breast milk. Often, the breasts are much more receptive to lactation--and sometimes produce more milk--in the morning, so if you are able to begin each day with a beautifully rejuvenating nursing session, that is fantastic! If not, don't worry. Remember, this schedule is meant to fit your needs, so select a time that's convenient for you.

This schedule works perfectly for someone who has not previously lactated as well as for women who have begun the journey of re-lactation. It is also helpful to post-menopausal women, and those who have undergone hysterectomies.

It also allows you to choose your level of lactation, which means that if you decide to become partially lactated, and then later opt to pursue full lactation, you can do so, simply by continuing to follow this schedule and adjusting the number of times you nurse in a 24-hour period.

Another beautiful factor is the 2.4-hour time window that this flexible nursing schedule provides. If you find that you truly aren't able to nurse at your set time, you will be able to nurse 2.4 hours prior to or 2.4 hours after your regularly scheduled nursing without fear of missing the opportunity to induce.

When using this schedule, you must be sure to nurse 9 out of every 10 days, which means that you will have to nurse 27 times in a

30-day period of time to ensure results.

When Mr. S and I committed to induce lactation, we nursed for the entire 30 days. Although every cycle provides a couple with three "free days" in which they can miss a nursing session, he and I chose to nurse on those days, too. I would suggest that you and your partner nurse consecutively for the first 30 days without taking a "free day" if at all possible, as the first month is very important to the inducing of lactation. It is what sets the rhythm for the female body and breasts.

Another tip to help boost that milk supply is to drink an 8-ounce glass of water 15-20 minutes before nursing; you should then drink at least 4 ounces of water following each nursing session to ensure that your body remains well hydrated.

This is the nursing schedule that Mr. S and I have used with incredible results. We have now followed this schedule for 10 months, but after just three months, I had reached full lactation. You can personalize it in a way that suits you. Here is what my husband and I devised:

LMM and Mr. S' Nursing Schedule

Set nursing time: 11:00 p.m.

Earliest time available to nurse: 8:45 p.m.

Latest time possible to nurse: 1:15 a.m.

It honestly is that simple!

If you follow the guidelines of this schedule as you employ the lactation inducing techniques that we will explore in the following chapters of this book, I am confident that you, too, will be producing breast milk sooner than you believed possible!

Chapter 2

Lactation Technique #1
The Art of Suckling

Now that you understand the process of lactation, and what you may expect as you reach new phases in the journey, have practiced putting your partner to the breast, and set a comfortable and flexible nursing schedule that you can easily commit to, the time has come to begin making that precious liquid gold--and choosing how you will do so. You may, of course, decide to incorporate a variety of techniques to encourage milk production and flow, but in doing so, consistency will remain key.

In many ways, lactation is an emotional process that begins by the woman's desire to produce breast milk. By telling your body what you want, and requesting your milk from your breasts, you have already begun the process of lactation. When your brain receives the signal that milk is needed, over time, your body will take part in the process to provide it. Your milk will not flow until your breasts release it. Your mind controls the nerves and muscles of the breast, and this intricate network will only release the milk if you are emotionally attuned to the inducing process.

The first step in successful lactation is training your body to understand and recognize the let-down reflex, which is stimulated by your deep emotions and the desire to provide milk, and heavily influenced by the visualization techniques and reflex cues that were discussed in the first section of this book. After you become accustomed to it, like any other natural reflex action that your body performs, the let-down reflex becomes automatic and requires less outside stimulus; if you do find that you are having trouble establishing lactation, add the visualization and reflex cue stimuli into your daily inducing technique once more.

As nature has designed, suckling will always be the best choice for inducing lactation, as the breasts require deep stimulation to produce breast milk. Although this can be achieved by using other techniques, no method produces greater results than a properly suckling mouth. Along with providing correct stimulation, suckling naturally works to release the hormones needed to produce breast milk. This is why you should nurse your partner as frequently as possible, particularly in the beginning stages of lactation when your body is growing accustomed to its new routine, and when doing so, ensure that he is properly latched and correctly suckling.

There is a fine balance between under-stimulation and over-stimulation of the breasts, and both are ineffective when it comes to milk production and flow. To ensure lactation, your partner should suckle from each breast for a minimum of 20 minutes. The let-down reflex is normally triggered within the first five minutes of stimulation, so it is ideal if he applies the short, rapid succession of 'pacifier sucks" to each breast upon latching, as this encourages the release of milk. He should then spend the remaining time of the nursing experience using the slow and steady suck and swallow rhythm that encourages the released milk to flow from the breasts and through the nipple.

Your partner may choose to remain on the breast for a period of 30 minutes, and this length of time is still very effective in the lactation process, as long as he remembers to trigger the let-down reflex upon initial latch. After 30 minutes, suckling becomes ineffective, as the breasts begin to shut down, slowing the lactation process. He can remain on the breast for longer periods of time, but remember, if he does, suckling will be for pleasure rather than for   production.

Regardless of the length of time your partner chooses to nurse, be certain that he remains on each breast for the same amount of time, and stay as close to your set nursing time as you possibly can.

Chapter 3

Lactation Technique #2
Manual Stimulation

Manual stimulation simply means that you--or your partner--will use your hands to massage your breasts to aid in the lactation process, and this milk-making technique, while very effective if suckling is not an option for any particular reason, truly requires a great deal of dedication and a carefully regulated schedule.

When it comes to producing breast milk, a woman's body does not identify the process as either maternal or non-maternal, which means that nursing an adult is very similar to breastfeeding a child; your body reacts to Lactogenesis and milk synthesis regardless of pregnancy and childbirth, responding to the supply and demand factor in breast milk production, which is why staying true to your daily routine is crucial to successful lactation. During manual stimulation, if you alter the length of time you massage your breasts, or miss even one expression, your body believes that you are weaning a child from the breast, and will begin to revert to its previous non-lactated condition by reversing the inducing process. This is both discouraging and frustrating, and you will have to incorporate several more sessions back into your daily routine to reach the lactation level you had achieved before the reversal occurred. The only way to prevent this from happening is to be certain that you do not miss a manual stimulation session.

The extraction of breast milk is known as expression, and when you induce lactation through consistent manual stimulation, you will be expressing your breasts, and requesting milk, even if you're not yet producing milk; this technique allows you to stimulate your breasts as if you are lactating. Essentially, you will be applying pressure to your lobules, squeezing the milk that is inside your ducts, and bringing it forward to your nipple. Manual stimulation also ensures that you are emptying your breasts, particularly the milk that is stored behind the nipple.

To apply this lactation technique, grasp your breast by curving your hand into a cradled C-position with your thumb on the top of your breast and your fingers beneath it, resting closely to the wall of the chest. Begin by firmly compressing, or squeezing, your breast, as if to draw milk out. As you continue to apply this pressure, which will cause the breast to take on a bit of a flattened appearance, move your breast forward in a firm stroking motion. Be sure not to slide your fingers over your breast; you must move the breast, sliding the skin along with it. As you stimulate, you should also be sure to massage the areola in a counter-clockwise motion to activate the ductal network that lies in a circular pattern beneath it.

You should massage each breast for 10-15 minutes, and you will need to do this each day, every 3-4 hours. You can manually stimulate one breast before shifting to the opposite side, or apply the technique to both breasts simultaneously; just be sure that each breast is stimulated for the same length of time to ensure the technique's effectiveness.

While nursing, you or your partner can add manual stimulation as he suckles, which helps to empty the breasts, or, if you have a breast pump, it is often very helpful to pump your breasts for an additional five minutes after you have finished the full 10-15 minutes of manual stimulation. A good breast pump provides rapid-pulsing stimulation of the areolar nerves, which is a wonderful way to activate lactation.

And, speaking of breast pumps, let's now further discuss our third milk-making method.

Chapter 4

Lactation Technique #3
Breast Pump Stimulation

A good breast pump can be a valuable tool for those women who hope to induce lactation, but simply don't have the time to massage their breasts every day of every week on a strictly regulated schedule that involves approximately eight manual sessions in a 24-hour period of time. While not as effective as suckling or hand expression, as this method of inducing doesn't quite provide the depth of stimulation as the previously discussed techniques, pumping to induce lactation can still be beneficial, and is a milk-making method that many women use with great success. Pumping allows great flexibility, as you decide how often you will employ this technique. Important things to remember, regardless of how often you choose to pump, is consistency (do not vary your daily set pumping time) and the length of time you pump during each session. You should pump each breast for 10-15 minutes. Once you are producing milk, you should continue to pump, even if the flow stops during the session. Pumping for the entire 10-15 minutes aids in properly emptying your breasts, which, of course, lets your body know that you need more milk.

There are many pump options available, and whether you select a manual or electric model will be dependent upon your personal preference and needs. If you are committed to inducing lactation, particularly with the goal of being fully lactated, you might want to consider investing in a double electric pump, as this can be utilized to collect breast milk once you have reached a stage of expression. The opportunity to pump both breasts simultaneously comes in quite handy, as many women are juggling lactation and everyday life. You'll be able to find many fantastic hospital-grade breast pumps on the market, and many of them offer a variety of stimulation modes, which is a wonderful way to encourage the let-down reflex and further milk flow.

Just as with suckling, the suction of a breast pump has very little to do with milk production, so using a great deal of force, as in setting your pump to a level of maximum suction in hope of producing more milk more quickly, is counterproductive, and can be extremely painful.It is stimulation that produces breast milk, and suction that collects it. Pump gently, and for no longer than 20 minutes per side. Because a pump is not always effective at fully emptying your breasts, attempt to hand express for an additional five minutes after each pumping session. Once you are fully lactated, a breast pump becomes much more reliable and efficient, and you will be able to decrease the number of sessions you perform each day when you have determined your personal lactation desires.

Every breast pump includes a flange (or flanges, if you purchase a double pump). These are sometimes referred to as breast shields, and are the curved cups that are placed on the breasts prior to pumping. Flanges are extremely important to the pumping process. They must fit properly and be used properly to ensure effectiveness. Every woman is unique, and the average flange only fits about 45 percent of the female population, so you may find that you need to purchase a different size that is suited for you. Breasts are also unique, even if they belong to the same woman, so it is not uncommon to find that you might need a different size flange for each breast.

A flange creates a seal around the areola, so it needs to fit snugly without pressing painfully into the breast. To test your flange, center your nipple into the cup's tunnel, and hold the shield against your breast, ensuring the rim completely encircles your areola. Very little pressure is needed; allow your pump to provide the suction for you. Once your flange is properly positioned, turn your pump on, adjusting the suction to your maximum comfort level. Your nipple should move freely and easily into the tunnel without pain or resistance. If you notice that it is compressed or rubs along the side of the flange tunnel, or there is any discoloration of the nipple or flesh of the breast, then your flange is probably too small. While testing your shield, if it feels loose around the edges, or you notice a pinching sensation as your nipple and areola are pulled into the tunnel, then, more than likely, your flange is too big, so be sure to adjust your breast shields accordingly, and before removing them from your breasts, be sure that you have turned off your pump's suction function to properly break the seal.

Perfecting the art of lactation requires a bit of trial and error, but once you have learned a few tricks of the trade, you will be a master milk maker in no time!

Chapter 5

Lactation Technique #4
TENS Unit Stimulation

A Transcutaneous Electrical Nerve Stimulation (TENS) Unit is a medical device comprised of channels and electrodes (pads). A TENS Unit produces a very low electrical micro-current that flows from one electrode (pad) of each unit channel to the other electrode of the same channel. A single channel unit contains one channel and two electrodes while a double unit is comprised of two channels and four electrodes. The original use of a TENS Unit was meant to stimulate the body's nerve in an effort to mask pain, but it's purpose in aiding lactation is to actively stimulate the nerves of the breast, particularly in the nipple and areola, in an effort to release prolactin and encourage milk production.

While it is not meant to replace more traditional forms of breast stimulation, such as suckling, hand expression, or pumping, the TENS Unit is increasing in popularity as an effective form of inducing lactation for the busy and active woman. The unit, which is very compact and lightweight, can be slipped into a bra or pocket, and because it produces no audible vibration or noise, it can be used discreetly while you're at work, running errand, or involved in any other day-to-day activity.

If you choose to induce lactation by using the TENS method, it is best to select a double channel unit so you will be able to conveniently stimulate both breasts simultaneously. The TENS unit relies on the skin of your breasts to act as an electrical conductor when the pads are in place; when it is turned on, you will feel a pleasant tingling sensation in the nipple and areola.

To properly use your TENS unit, stand in

front of a mirror and use one channel for your left breast and the second channel for your right breast. The pads will be marked to identify a positive (+) electrode and a negative (-) electrode. Beginning with your left breast, apply the positive electrode pad to your breast, approximately one inch from the side of your nipple, and then apply the negative pad directly across from it, one inch from the opposite side of your nipple. Repeat this process with the second channel, placing the pads on either side of your right nipple. When looking in the mirror, the unit's channels, electrodes, and your nipples should be well-aligned, and it should look something like this:

+Electrode (breast) Left nipple (breast) -Electrode (cleavage) -Electrode (breast) Right Nipple (breast) +Electrode, or:

(+ o -)| (- o +), which signifies the proper

electrode placement and alignment, when looking in a mirror.

Once the pads are in place, you can get dressed, and begin stimulation simply by turning on the unit, which can be used every two hours for 15 minutes throughout the day. After 15 minutes, stimulation to induce lactation becomes ineffective, as the breasts shut down the release of prolactin, further impeding the milk-making process.

Your TENS Unit may be equipped with a variety of mode options, and below are a few setting suggestions that you may find helpful:

Wave Form: Choose the form that is indicative of massage.

Amplitude: Use this to adjust the current, setting it low to create a light tingling in the nipples and areolae.

Pulse Width: This function determines how long each pulse lasts, and should be set in a manner that is comparable to that of an infant's suction, which is normally half of a second in length; you can set the width to the longest possible pulse, which is 250 us.

Frequency: This setting is used to determine how often your breast will be stimulated while the TENS in use, and should also closely compare to the rate of an infant's suckling mouth, so set this to 70.

It is important to note that although quite useful in helping to stimulate the breasts, a TENS Unit cannot empty the breasts, which is why utilizing another preferred method of milk removal is necessary when using this method of stimulation. The unit also has no way of collecting expressed breast milk, and once you have begun to produce, the TENS vibrations will cause your milk to flow, which means wet bras and blouses, so consider this carefully and plan accordingly.

A final, and very important note, concerning the use of a TENS Unit is a matter of heart health and physical well-being. The amperage of an electrical current can cause heart arrhythmia, although most physicians agree that, because TENS units have a very small micro-amperage current, it would be unlikely that the device would cause problems for most women, concurring that it is safer to use a double channel unit with four pads, placing two electrodes on each breast, rather than a single channel unit, as this allows the current to travel through the electrodes rather than through the chest. If you have an implanted pacemaker or defibrillator, you should not use a TENS Unit.

As always, it is best to consult your health care provider with health concerns and safety issues. He or she will be able to answer any questions that you may have regarding the personal use of a TENS Unit, and help you decide if the device is right for you.

Chapter 6

Power Pumping

Power pumping is an inducing technique that encourages the breasts to produce more milk at an increased rate by mimicking the frequent nursing of an infant who is experiencing a growth spurt. At this time in an infant's life, he or she will often suckle more frequently, more vigorously, and for longer periods of time, which triggers an increased release of prolactin from the pituitary gland, sending the "make more milk more quickly" message to the nursing woman's breasts.

To effectively power pump, begin by choosing one hour every day (for example, 8 a.m.), and then follow this pumping pattern:

1.Pump for 20 minutes. Rest for 10 minutes.

2.Pump for another 10 minutes. Rest for 10 minutes.

3.Pump an additional 10 minutes. Finish.

This provides 40 minutes of pumping in a 60 minute period of time. Throughout the day, you should continue using your other lactation inducing techniques (suckling, hand expression, traditional pumping, and/or TENS stimulation) to help the process along. Many women find that implementing this technique on three consecutive days is sufficient in increasing their milk supply while others choose to power pump for longer periods of time, typically seven consecutive days.

Most women see an increase in their milk supply 48 hours to one week after they begin their power pump routine, but don't be discouraged if your body responds a bit slower to this lactation technique. Perseverance and consistency are key factors in this milk making method.

To use an alternative method of the technique dubbed "Power Pumping Boot Camp", you can perform four of these sessions each day for two days before resuming your regular pumping routine. Because proper rest is vital to breast milk production, you should not set an alarm to wake you to pump through the night.

Clock-watching and alarm-setting to be certain that you are power pumping for the proper amount of time is stressful, and stress impedes milk production, so get comfortable and relax as you pump by watching your favorite movie and pumping during one scene before resting during the next, or enjoying a television show and pumping through the commercials. You can even put on a favorite CD and pump while listening to two songs before resting through the next two.

To effectively power pump, it is best to use a good quality medical-grade electric breast pump, which handles this lactation inducing technique much more quickly and efficiently than a manual pump, as you can set functions and cycles to closely mimic the suckling patterns of a growing infant.

No matter the inducing method you use, always remember to be persistent and patient. Your desired level of lactation awaits--it may simply take some time to get there!

Chapter 7

The Marmet Technique

One of the earliest writings on the Marmet Technique, a form of manual expression used to drain the breast milk reservoirs, was published in 1978 by Chele Marmet and the Lactation Institute of Ventura, California, and some women are now using this as a form of inducing lactation.

Here are instructions on utilizing this technique:

1. Position the thumb (above the nipple) and first two fingers (below the nipple) about 1" to 1–1/2" from the nipple, though not necessarily at the outer edges of the areola. Use this measurement as a guide, since breasts and areolae vary in size from one woman to another. Be sure the hand forms the letter "C" and the finger pads are at 6 and 12 o'clock in

line with the nipple.

• Avoid cupping the breast

2. Push straight into the chest wall

• Avoid spreading the fingers apart.

• For large breasts, first lift and then push into the chest wall

3. Roll thumb and fingers forward at the same time. This rolling motion compresses and empties milk reservoirs without injuring sensitive breast tissue.

4. Repeat rhythmically to completely drain reservoirs.

• Position, push, roll...

• Position, push, roll...

5. Rotate the thumb and fingers to milk other reservoirs, using both hands on each breast.

Avoid These Motions

1. Do not squeeze the breast, as this can cause bruising.

2. Sliding hands over the breast may cause

painful skin burns.

3. Pulling the nipple may result in tissue damage.

While many women find the Marmet Technique beneficial, it is best to employ this milk-making method with other forms of inducing throughout the day for greater success.

Chapter 8

Areola Massage to Aid in Lactation

In order to help assist the lactation process along, the breasts require deep and consistent stimulation. The best form of this stimulation is produced by a properly suckling mouth, but if your partner is unavailable to come to the breast for a nursing session, manual, or hand, stimulation is a wonderful alternative. Many women prefer to use a breast pump in their partner's absence, and while this is a perfectly acceptable choice to aid in stimulation, a pump really doesn't provide the depth of stimulation required to help with milk production and flow in the beginning of the lactation process. Even before you are producing breast milk, you need to express your breasts as if you are lactating to let them know that there is a need for that beautiful milk.

Areola stimulation is a terrific way to get those milk ducts contracting, and this inducing technique can be done alone, or with your partner prior to nursing.

Nestled within the areolae in a circular pattern is a network of nerves and tiny muscles that, when stimulated, send signals to your breasts--and brain--that encourages your body to begin the process of milk production. During breast massage, be sure to focus on the entire breast, paying particular attention to the areola.

To manually express your breasts (even if you aren't yet producing breast milk) using this method of stimulation, simply cover your areola with the flattened palm of your hand, fingers pointing down, and center your nipple against your palm. Press inward firmly, pulling your breast against the wall of the chest, and begin to massage the areola in a smooth, circular counter-clockwise motion. Be sure to move your breast rather than your hand while performing this stimulation technique. Your grip should provide smooth, firm pressure, but never any pain.

You can apply this technique to both breasts simultaneously, or stimulate each breast individually. When using areola stimulation, be sure to massage each breast for a full 10-15 minutes every 3-4 hours.

Remember: it is perfectly fine to incorporate a variety of inducing techniques into your daily routine! As a matter of fact, I recommend it. There's no better way to get that breast milk flowing! No matter what techniques you use, be sure to nurse as frequently as you can, and definitely during your set nursing times!

Chapter 9

Breast Compressions to Encourage Milk Flow while Nursing

Breast compressions are a wonderful way to encourage milk flow, and are very helpful during the suckling experience to ensure that your partner is consuming every drop of breast milk you make and properly emptying your breasts during each nursing session, which helps greatly in the lactation process by telling your body that more milk is needed. Although they do very little to assist in the process of making milk, these compressions cam help with flow. They are effective during suckling, and while they can be used during any level of lactation, they are particularly useful during the first phase of inducing or re-lactation when milk supply is low, and it is sometimes difficult to tell precisely how much milk you're releasing during each nursing session. Breast compressions can also be helpful if your milk flow has slowed, or your partner isn't suckling effectively.

Here's how to put the squeeze on lactation.

Once you and your partner have settled into a comfortable nursing position and he is properly latched to the breast, allow him to suckle for approximately five minutes to encourage the let-down reflex. You can then incorporate your first set of breast compressions.

To provide proper compressions, curve your hand into a C-shape, allowing the side of your breast to rest comfortably in the cupped palm of your hand with your fingers supporting the underside of the breast and resting against the wall of the chest. Your thumb will lie flat along the top of the areola, and help to provide pressure during this technique. Your thumb should not press into the areola, as this can inhibit milk flow; when performing compressions, be sure not to disturb your partner's latch. If he does come off the breast, help him re-latch, and then re-position your hand. Firmly squeeze your breast. Your fingers will push upward while your thumb presses down, and the breast will flatten slightly. Hold the position for five minutes as your partner suckles, then release. The release allows your hand and breast to rest. Your partner should continue to nurse during this rest. After five minute have gone by, apply a second five-minute set of breast compressions if you wish, and repeat the process (compress-rest) for the length of the entire nursing session. You can compress either one or both breasts.

Compressions is a technique that don't require a great deal of consistency, so you don't need to use them during every nursing session, as skipping compressions will not adversely affect breast milk production in any way.

I have used breast compressions many times during nursing sessions, and have always found them to be very helpful! There are times when Mr. S isn't sure that he has completely emptied my breasts, so he or I simply perform a set of compressions, and we can be sure that we're encouraging a fabulous supply of milk.

٭

Chapter 10

How to Use a Manual Breast Pump to Maximize Efficiency and Effectiveness

There is a wide selection of breast pumps available on the market, and nursing women have very discerning tastes when it comes to their particular pump of choice, often going to great lengths to find one that is perfectly suited to their particular needs. I found myself facing that same dilemma early into my non-maternal lactation journey. If you've read some of my earlier posts on my website, you'll know that, as a breastfeeding mother, I wasn't a huge breast pump fan, and I wasn't sure that I was going to pump within my ANR. I soon discovered, however, that pumping was actually going to be a necessity, so I began to look into pump options. I first chose a single manual pump before investing in a hospital-grade electric pump.

There is a lot of debate over the manual versus electric pump. Although electric pumps can be a lot more convenient for in-home use, they aren't always practical for active non-maternal nursing women on the go. Adult nursing is a private and discreet part of many couple's lives, and explaining why you're carrying an electric breast pump with you when there are obviously no little ones to sustain is simply not a viable option. Manual pumps take care of that problem; they are lightweight, easy to assemble, and can be discreetly stored away from prying eyes. And they are also much more economical than their electric counterparts.

Electric breast pumps can be expensive, ranging from about $179.00 upwards to $500.00 or more--an this price doesn't include a carrying case. The cost of investing in an electric breast pump just isn't in everyone's budget.

I do love my electric breast pump; it does a lot of the work for me, as I can efficiently pump both breasts at once, and set the controls to determine let-down stimulation, suckling stimulation, and my maximum comfort level, but, with that being said, I also found that my manual pump was a true lifesaver early on, and I'm really glad that I had it on hand. It did its job very well, and has actually worked quite well to collect milk now that I am fully lactated and actively producing.

I would suggest that women new to ANR first invest in a manual pump; you can sort of "test the waters" to determine if you'll enjoy pumping before making a very large purchase. Later, as you commit to the pumping process, begin to require more stimulation, or after you have begun to produce larger quantities of milk, you may want to consider investing in an electric model. To get started, a manual pump is really all that you'll need.

While it's true that breast pumps can provide very good stimulation to help with milk production, their main goal is actually to draw milk from the breast and collect it. That's why using a pump to encourage lactation needs to be done properly. Essentially, you want your breasts to believe that there is a need for all of that beautiful milk, and the best way to do that is to mimic the feeding pattern of an infant. You can do this easily with a manual breast pump.

Before I explain how to do this, I thought I would share a few tips with you.

1. Flange (or breast shield) size is very important. The rim of your shield needs to completely encircle your areola. If you have large breasts, you'll notice that there is quite a bit of uncovered breast on either side of the flange. (Mr. S and I tease, calling it "overspill" or "excess boobage") Don't worry--as long as

your areola is covered, you'll be just fine.

Your flange should not compress your breast by squeezing or pinching it; there should be no pain at all. You should only feel a deep pull against the breast.

Your flange should not pull your areola or excess breast tissue into it, either. Once you have centered your nipple into the flange tunnel, it should move freely forward--and it should be the only part of your breast inside that tunnel.

2. Suction is another important part of using a manual pump properly. Some women pump harshly, and well over their maximum comfort level, believing that the forceful stimulation is necessary to efficient milk production. It isn't. Remember, vacuum is only used to collect breast milk; it really has nothing to do with making breast milk.

Something to avoid:

My breast shield always feels too tight,

and I have trouble taking it off of my breast. I've been using Vaseline, and now, it slides right off.

A breast shield should fit snugly. If it feels too tight, as if its squeezing your breast, then it is probably either too small or you are pumping with too much force.

Petroleum jelly can damage the materials used to make breast shields, so I wouldn't suggest using it as a lubricant. It's important to remember to break your pump's suction before removing a flange from your breast. If you still feel that a lubricant is necessary, though, coconut oil is a better choice. It won't break down your flange, and it's very good for your breasts.

Most manual pumps are equipped with some sort of device (a lever or a button) that allows a woman to adjust the tension and resistance of her pump handle, which helps to either simulate the let-down reflex or suckling.

My Lansinoh manual pump has a small white lever on the top of the handle; by sliding it back, I can simulate let-down. To trigger let-down, adjust your pump to its highest resistance level before you begin. When you do this, the handle will tighten.

On a manual pump, maximum comfort level is typically determined by how a woman depresses her pump handle. If you press the handle "all the way" into the pump's collection bottle, sometimes hearing the click of the contact, the suction will be much more forceful, and you will be pumping at maximum level. You don't need to do this unless you want to; your pump will work just as effectively if you only depress the handle halfway in. It isn't the force of the pumping, but the rhythm of the motions that is important.

When first put to the breast, an infant sucks very rapidly to encourage milk flow. These quick "pacifier sucks" offer no pause for a "swallow rest". Infants provide two sucks per second when attempting to trigger let-down.

To mimic this rhythm with your manual pump, you will need to depress the handle in quick, short repeated bursts. You can do this by counting "1-2, 1-2, 1-2" to easily time the rhythm. It will be a continuous motion, fast, but steady, and you'll need to repeat this for 3-5 minutes to ensure that let-down has occurred.

Manual pumps provide "comfort grip handles" to prevent hand and arm fatigue, but when you first begin manual pumping, no matter how "comfortable" that handle is, you'll feel the effects. It's strenuous to pump, but it gets a lot easier as your hands adapt to the motion. It's important to keep up that fast "1-2" let-down motion when pumping, but if you can't do it for five minutes without breaking, stop and rest for a minute or two, before picking up your rhythm once more. Just remember, the rest time doesn't count as active pumping time, so be sure to actively pump for 3-5 minutes.

When you have triggered let-down, you can adjust your pump's tension to simulate proper suckling. When I slide my pump's lever forward, the tension loosens and my handle becomes much easier to depress.

When a baby realizes that the time to actually eat has arrived, he slows his suckling to a content and leisurely rate, pausing to swallow in between sucks. Babies are so attuned to the breast that they will actually adjust their feeding rhythm to ensure maximum efficiency. They will often show a ratio of two sucks for every one swallow, or even three sucks per swallow.

To pattern this suck-swallow rhythm while using your manual pump, you will do this by depressing and then releasing your pump's handle. The two depresses represent "suck-suck", and the rest release represents "swallow". You can time the rhythm by repeating "1,2-rest...1-2-rest..." or "1-2-3-rest" as you pump. The depressions will be rapid; just as with let-down stimulation, you will still depress the handle twice (or even three times) per second, but the rest will last for approximately two seconds.

You will need to continue this pattern for about 10-15 minutes, depending on the length of time you pumped to simulate let-down.

Be sure to pump each breast in the same way, for the same length of time to ensure proper stimulation.

Before you know it, you'll be a breast pumping pro!

Part III

Supplements and Super Foods

Chapter 1

Herbal Supplements to Aid in Lactation

A galactogogue, or lactogenic, is an herb or other substance, such as a prescription medication, that is used to help increase breast milk supply, and even improve the let-down reflex, in nursing women, and the decision to add herbal supplements into your daily lactation routine is a very personal one. For some women, herbs are a feasible option when hoping to encourage a swifter increase in breast milk supply, and, after a bit of deliberation, others may decide that herbs are not really right for them. There is currently a lactation product on the market that proclaims to be a "miracle in a bottle", which is quite misleading to women who long to lactate. While it would be wonderful to have access to such a product, there is simply no miraculous or magical means of making more breast milk, and herbal supplements hold very stark realities. While they can aid in the lactation process, they will not simply make milk for you. Herbs and other lactogenic food sources simply help the process along, and taking them will require you to continue the use of applicable lactation techniques, such as suckling, hand expression, pumping, and TENS stimulation, and some women find that these methods remain more effective than taking supplements.

That is not to say that there is no success to be found from including lactogenic herbs (and nature's other finest super foods, which I myself use with fantastic results) in your lactation routine. There is, and many women have achieved wonderful results from the incorporation of herbs. Opinions and results vary greatly, of course, and it's very important to remember that not every woman will respond to herbal supplements in the same way, or in the same length of time.

Before we explore some of the most effective, and often commonly used, galactogogues, let's discuss what is already known about every herb.

1. Herbs may be carefully packaged and stamped as "organically certified", but they are not FDA approved or regulated, and while they may have been prepared in a FDA-registered facility, this does not mean that they are FDA-certified.

2. Even though they are natural, herbs should be used with caution, as you can suffer allergic reactions upon consumption, and even "overdose" if they are not consumed properly.

3. Herbs do have side effect warnings.

4. Herbs can negatively affect prescription medications, as they do carry drug interaction warnings with them.

5. Many herbs are not recommended for women who are pregnant or currently nursing.

6. Herbal supplements can pass through breast milk, which means that your partner will be taking them, too.

7. It is important that you always check with a health care professional prior to beginning any herbal regimen.

The FDA does play some role in the production, marketing, and sale of all herbs, but they handle them as a food rather than as a medication, so their medicinal effectiveness is not proven or guaranteed to consumers.

While "fresh is usually best", when it comes to choosing an herbal galactagogue, it is better to opt for a dried root, leaf, flower, or seed, particularly if you will be using them as a tea or infusion. The process of drying fresh herbs locks in their medicinal, nutritive, and lactogenic properties, which leads to their effectiveness as galactagogues.

If you have been taking an herbal galactagogue for several weeks without achieving noticeable results in your milk supply, you might want to check your supplement for freshness. Dried herbs have very good color and distinct aromas. If the color of your herb seems dull or "faded", or has lost a lot of its color and smell, it is probably old, and old herbs lose their effectiveness. Try replacing it with a new supply, and see if you notice an improvement.

Over time, and with repeated use, our bodies begin to adapt to new routines, and naturally build a tolerance for, or even a resistance to, certain medications; herbal supplements are no exception to this, and may attribute to a particular galactagogue's seemingly ineffective properties. If you have been using a lactogenic herb for several weeks without noticing results, your body may have built up an immunity to it. Try switching to a different lactogenic source, or combining a variety of galactagogues, to see if this helps.

Storing dried herbs in a glass airtight container with a well-fitting lid is the best way to preserve freshness, flavor, and nutritive properties. Placing them in a cool, dark, dry place will keep them fresh for a minimum of 18 months.

Please note that the herbs listed on the following pages of this guide are often used to aid in many health issues (ranging from diabetes and heart disease to digestive problems and kidney disorders), so I will not be focusing solely on their lactation properties, and because there are drug interaction warnings associated with these herbs, and the list is fairly extensive and not all-inclusive, I have used terms such as "some" and "several" as a generalization; you will need to check with your physician to ensure that a particular herb is right for you. If you are currently taking a prescription medication that is not listed beneath each medication interaction heading, it is recommended that you speak with a qualified health care professional to be sure that combining your medication with a galactagogue is safe for you. Although some herbs are commonly listed here, and in other herbal resources, as safe for pregnant women, always use your own judgment when taking any herbal supplement, as many are estrogenic and highly hormonal, particularly if you are at a risk for miscarriage.

There are many other lactogenics available, of course, which I explore in my book, *A Garden of Gold,* but these may help you as you begin the exploration of incorprating herbal supplements into your daily inducing routine.

1. Alfalfa

(Medicago sativa)

Alfalfa is a perennial flowering plant in the pea family, often cultivated as an important forage crop in many countries around the world. It is used for grazing, hay, and silage. While the name alfalfa is used in North America, the plant is commonly known as lucerne in the United Kingdom, South Africa, Australia, and New Zealand. In appearance, alfalfa resembles clover, with clusters of small purple flowers followed by spiraling fruits that contain 10–20 seeds. Alfalfa is native to warmer temperate climates, and has been cultivated as livestock fodder since the era of the ancient Greeks and Romans.

Alfalfa is said to promote the development of the glandular tissue of the breasts. It increases both milk supply and the fat content of breast milk, and is traditionally prescribed to promote the function of the pituitary gland, the source of the main hormones for lactation, and is one of our most nutritious herbs, and is a great choice for increasing breast milk production, as it is highly nutritious, easy to absorb, and rich in chlorophyll, a host of minerals, such as calcium, magnesium, phosphorus, potassium, silicon, and zinc, and vitamins A, B1, B2, B3, B5, B6, C, D, E, and K, as well as essential and non-essential amino acids.

Non-Lactogenic Uses:

Alfalfa is thought to lower total cholesterol and "bad" low-density lipoprotein (LDL) cholesterol in people with high cholesterol levels, and is also used to treat those who suffer from kidney, bladder, and prostate problems, asthma, arthritis, diabetes, and can even help with upset stomach.

Warnings:

Because alfalfa is a powerful galactagogue, it is important to decrease--or even discontinue--the use of alfalfa if oversupply of breast milk is noted.

Allergies:

You should not use alfalfa if you are allergic to peanuts and/or legumes.

Pregnancy Information:

Although an estrogenic herb that can be taken to promote menstruation, alfalfa is thought to be relatively safe when taken during pregnancy. However, be sure not to exceed the maximum recommended dosage, and to be certain that alfalfa is a safe choice for you, consult your doctor before taking it.

Health Precautions:

Although alfalfa is relatively safe for most adults, taking this herb for an extended period of time or in a dose larger than what is suggested is not recommended, as the herb can cause reactions that are similar to the autoimmune disease lupus.

Because of its high levels of Vitamin K, which helps blood to clot, it is not recommended for people who suffer from blood disorders. Warfarin (Coumadin) is used to slow blood clotting; alfalfa might decrease the effectiveness of this medication, so it is important that your blood is checked regularly, as the dose of your Warfarin might need to be adjusted.

Side Effects:

Because alfalfa contains photosynthesizing properties, it may cause some people to become extra-sensitive to sunlight, which can cause burning, blistering, or skin rash. Be sure to take precaution when outdoors by wearing sunblock and protective clothing.

Medication Interactions:

Alfalfa is believed to aid in helping the immune system's overall function, which can sometimes cause an increase in the symptoms associated with certain auto-immune diseases such as multiple sclerosis, lupus, and rheumatoid arthritis, and may negatively interact with some immunosuppressants. If you are currently taking azathioprine (Imuran), basiliximab (Simulect), cyclosporine (Neoral, Sandimmune), daclizumab (Zenapax), muromonab-CD3 (OKT3, Orthoclone OKT3), mycophenolate (CellCept), tacrolimus (FK506, Prograf), sirolimus (Rapamune), prednisone (Deltasone, Orasone), corticosteroids (glucocorticoids), or any other immunosuppressant, be sure to talk to your doctor before taking alfalfa.

Some medications can increase sensitivity to sunlight, and large doses of alfalfa might also increase your sensitivity to sunlight. Taking alfalfa along with photosensitive medications, such as amitriptyline (Elavil), Ciprofloxacin (Cipro), norfloxacin (Noroxin), lomefloxacin (Maxaquin), ofloxacin (Floxin), levofloxacin (Levaquin), sparfloxacin (Zagam), gatifloxacin (Tequin), moxifloxacin (Avelox), trimethoprim/sulfamethoxazole (Septra), tetracycline, methoxsalen (8-methoxypsoralen,

8-MOP, Oxsoralen), and Trioxsalen (Trisoralen), may increase your risk of sunburn, blistering, or rashes on areas of skin exposed to sunlight, so bee sure to take precautions by wearing sunblock and protective clothing when spending time outdoors.

Alfalfa might lower blood sugar levels, so if you have diabetes and take alfalfa, monitor your blood sugar levels closely.

Because alfalfa may have some of the same effects as estrogen, conjugated equine estrogens (Premarin), ethinyl estradiol, and estradiol may negatively interact with this supplement. It is important to remember that many birth control pills, such as ethinyl estradiol and levonorgestrel (Triphasil), ethinyl estradiol and norethindrone (Ortho-Novum 1/35, Ortho-Novum 7/7/7), contain estrogen, and because alfalfa may decrease the contraceptive's effectiveness, you may want to use an additional form of birth control while taking alfalfa.

Dosage and Preparation:

As a tea: Add one to two teaspoons of dried alfalfa to one cup of water. Drink up to three cups of tea per day. (To kick-start milk supply, drink up to six cups of tea per day for several days. An increase in milk supply may be noticeable within two to four days.)

Infusion method: Add one to two handfuls of dried alfalfa to one quart jar of boiling water. Cover tightly, and allow to steep for 10 hours, or over night, before consuming.

As a supplement: Up to 60 grams daily in capsule form.

2. Anise

(Pimpinella anisum)

Sometimes known as aniseed, anise is a flowering herbaceous annual plant native to the eastern Mediterranean region and Southwest Asia, first cultivated in Egypt and the Middle East, but then brought to Europe for its medicinal purposes. Anise plants grow three foot or more in height, and the 3/8-2-inch leaves at the base of the plant are very simple, long and shallowly lobed, while leaves higher on the stems are feathery pinnate, divided into several small leaflets. The flowers are white, approximately 1/8 inch in diameter, and the fruit, normally referred to as aniseed, is dry and oblong with flavor very similar to fennel and black licorice, which is why many Western cuisines have long used this herb to flavor a variety of dishes, drinks, and candies.

Anise is an umbel seed, which can be blended with other umbel seeds to maximize their effectiveness as a galactagogue. Every umbrel seed is estrogenic and promote relaxation, as they act as a natural sedative, supports digestion, and act as an anti-spasmodic to aid in treating bronchitis and bronchial asthma.

Non-Lactogenic Uses:

Along with helping to increase breast milk supply, anise is often used to treat discomforts brought on by a woman's menstrual cycle, asthma, certain sleep disorders, coughs, and some skin conditions, such as psoriasis. It can even aid to increase the human sex drive. While believed to be a relatively safe herb for most healthy adults who follow proper dosing suggestions, anise can exacerbate certain medical conditions and negatively interact with some medications.

Warnings:

Do not confuse this herb with Japanese star anise, which is toxic.

Allergies:

Anise might cause allergic reactions in some people who suffer from allergies to asparagus, caraway, celery, coriander, cumin, dill, and fennel.

Pregnancy Information:

Anise is listed as unsafe during pregnancy.

Because it has been used in traditional medicine to promote menstruation, it is believed that anise could trigger miscarriage. Do not use anise while pregnant.

Health Precautions:

Hormone-sensitive condition such as breast cancer, uterine cancer, ovarian cancer, endometriosis, or uterine fibroids, made worse by the exposure to estrogen, may be negatively affected by anise.

Side Effects:

There are no known side effects associated with the use of anise.

Medication Interactions:

Do not take anise if you are currently taking tamoxifen (Nolvadex).

Because of its etrogenic properties, anise may decrease the effectiveness of some birth control pills, such as ethinyl estradiol and levonorgestrel (Triphasil), ethinyl estradiol and norethindrone (Ortho-Novum 1/35, and

Ortho-Novum 7/7/7), and may adversely affect estrogen pills, including conjugated equine estrogens (Premarin), ethinyl estradiol, and estradiol.

Dosage and Preparation:

As a tea: Gently crush one to two teaspoons of anise seeds, and cover with one cup of boiling water. Cover and steep for five to 20 minutes. Sweeten to taste. Drink three cups of tea per day. (To kick start milk production, drink up to six cups of anise tea for two to four days.

Infusion method: Place one cup of anise seeds in a quart jar of boiling water. Cover and allow to steep for a minimum of four hours before consuming.

As a tincture: 3.5 to 7 grams daily.

3. Blessed Thistle

(Cnicus benedictus)

Blessed Thistle, sometimes known as "Our Lady's Milk Thistle", is as its name suggests, a thistle-like annual plant, native to the Mediterranean region, from Portugal in the north north to southern France, and east to Iran. It is known in other parts of the world, too, including certain regions of North America, as an introduced species of plant, and often, a noxious weed. Blessed Thistle generally grows to approximately well over one foot in height, with leathery, spine-covered leaves measuring one-half foot long and approximately 3 5/8 inches wide. The yellow flowers are produced in a flowerhead surrounded by many spiny basal bracts. While not typically considered edible, the leaves, flowers, and stems of Blessed Thistle is often used as a galactagogue to promote lactation and as a compound within some medicinal bitters. The use of Blessed Thistle dates back to the Middle Ages when it was used to treat the bubonic plague and given as a tonic of health to monks. This herb in tincture form is even mentioned as a cure for the common cold in William Shakespeare's play, *Much Ado about Nothing*.

Blessed thistle increases the flow of gastric and bile secretion, and is used in the treatment of stomach, intestines, liver, and gall bladder disease as a digestive bitter. Remember that bitter teas need to taste bitter in order to trigger the release of gastric juices and stimulate the production of bile, so do not over-sweeten this tea.

Non-Lactogenic Uses:

Along with healing wounds and promoting breast milk flow, Blessed Thistle is also often used to treat diarrhea, coughs, and infections, and while believed to be relatively safe for most healthy adults, using larger quantities of the recommended daily dosage of Blessed Thistle, generally set at five grams per cup of tea, may cause stomach irritation and vomiting. People who suffer from intestinal problems, such as Crohn's disease, infection, and other inflammatory disorders of the stomach should avoid using Blessed Thistle.

Allergies:

This herb may also cause allergic reactions in people who have allergies to ragweed, chrysanthemums, marigolds, and daisies.

Pregnancy Information:

Blessed thistle should not be taken during pregnancy.

Health Precautions:

Blessed thistle may exacerbate some medical conditions and intestinal problems, such as infections, Crohn's disease, and other inflammatory conditions by further irritating the stomach and intestine.

Side Effects:

Blessed thistle may cause vomiting if taken in excess.

Medication Interactions:

Because Blessed Thistle can increase the amount of acid in the stomach, it can adversely affect over the counter antacids such as Tums and Rol-Aids, which often contain calcium carbonate and sodium carbonate, and presription medications known as H2-Blockers, that may include cimetidine (Tagamet), ranitidine (Zantac), nizatidine (Axid), and famotidine (Pepcid) as well as proton pump inhibitors.

Dosage and Preparation:

As a tea: Pour a cup of boiling water over one to two teaspoons of dried blessed thistle. Steep for minutes. Drink three cups of tea per day, before meals or snacks. (To kick-start lactation, you may drink up to five cups of tea per day.)

As a supplement: Up to 2 grams daily in capsule form.

Combination Suggestion:

Blessed thistle can be taken in conjunction with fenugreek.

4. Fenugreek

(Trigonella foenum-graecum)

As one of the oldest plants cultivated for its medicinal properties and native to southern Europe and Asia, Fenugreek is now grown in the Mediterranean countries, Argentina, France, India, North Africa, and the United States, as a food, condiment, medicinal, dye, and forage plant. An annual herb similar to clover, the plant is identified by its three teardrop-shaped leaves and white flowers that appear in the early summer and develop into slim tan pods that contain brown seeds.

While Fenugreek seeds contain hormone precursors that increase breast milk supply, scientists still aren't clear why this happens. Some theorize that it may occur because breasts are modified sweat glands and

Fenugreek is known to stimulate sweat production. It has been shown that Fenugreek can increase a nursing woman's breast milk supply within 24-72 hours, and that once an adequate lactation level has been achieved, most women can discontinue taking the herb and maintain their supply with proper breast stimulation and milk removal.

Fenugreek has long been known to be effective as a natural breast enlarger, as the herb's diosgenin are used to make synthetic estrogen that has been shown to cause growth in breast cells. The herb may also help to increase sexual desire and improve the breasts' overall beauty and health. Fenugreek also contains choline, which may aid in the thinking process, and antioxidants that slow aging and help to prevent disease.

Fenugreek also has the keen ability to produce a maple syrup scent, which is a normal and to-be-expected side effect; as a matter of fact, when you (or your partner) begin to notice this sweet, syrup-y scent (which can be detected in perspiration, other bodily fluids, and even in breast milk), you'll know that you have reached the adequate dosage of Fenugreek.

Fenugreek contains a very potent aromatic compound called solotone, which can be found in lovage (an edible plant from the parsley family), aged rums, and molasses. Solotone passes through the body, and when consumed in large quantities, can prompt the "maple syrup effect".

Though most women respond quickly to fenugreek seed tea, capsules, or tincture, not all do. Some see more success when taking fenugreek in combination with other lactogenic herbs. If you do not respond well to fenugreek, open a capsule to check the freshness and quality of the powdered herb, which should have a distinct color and smell. If it does not, the herb may be old and may have lost its therapeutic effect. Buying a fresher product may solve the problem.

Non-Lactogenic Uses:

Fenugreek is taken for digestive problems such as loss of appetite, upset stomach, constipation, and gastritis; it can be used for diabetes, painful menstruation, polycystic ovary syndrome, and obesity, atherosclerosis, and to treat both high cholesterol and triglycerides. Other uses include kidney ailments, mouth ulcers, boils, bronchitis, cellulitis, tuberculosis, chronic coughs, chapped lips, baldness, cancer, Parkinson's disease, and exercise performance.

Warnings:

Fenugreek must be taken consistently to avoid a decrease in breast milk supply.

Allergies:

People who are allergic to soybeans, peanuts, legumes, and green peas might experience an allergic reaction to fenugreek.

Pregnancy Information:

Fenugreek should not be used during pregnancy.

Health Precautions:

Fenugreek can cause hypoglycemia, and should only be used under medical supervision if you are diabetic, or are currently taking any blood-thinning medications.

Side Effects:

Along with its distinct maple syrup aroma, fenugreek may cause diarrhea, stomach upset, bloating, and gas. Unless a person experiences hypersensitivity to this herb, these side effects typically disappear within a few days after the dosage has begun.

Medication Interactions

Fenugreek may adversely affect glimepiride (Amaryl), glyburide (DiaBeta, Glynase PresTab, Micronase), insulin, pioglitazone (Actos), rosiglitazone (Avandia), chlorpropamide

(Diabinese), glipizide (Glucotrol), and tolbutamide (Orinase), and may negatively interact with aspirin, clopidogrel (Plavix), diclofenac (Voltaren, Cataflam, others), ibuprofen (Advil, Motrin, others), naproxen (Anaprox, Naprosyn, others), dalteparin (Fragmin), enoxaparin (Lovenox), and heparin.

If you currently take Warfarin (Coumadin), check with your doctor to see if combining your medication with the use of fenugreek is safe for you.

Dosage and Preparation:

As a supplement: Take one fenugreek capsule the first day to see if you have an allergic reaction. If you do not have a reaction, then take three capsules the next day, dividing this amount in three doses, taken just before meals. Build the dosage slowly, adding one capsule per day, until you have reached the recommended standard daily dose of nine capsules. Gauge your reaction to the capsules carefully. Some women see a good improvement in their milk supply by taking only two capsules per day.

As a tea: Fenugreek seed can be adjusted to be either mild and delicate or potent and bitter, depending on how many seeds are added to water, and how long they are steeped. Pour eight ounces of boiling water over one to three teaspoons of fenugreek seeds and allow to steep for five to 10 minutes, or longer, before drinking. Sweeten to taste.

Cold Infusion: Place one cup of fenugreek seeds in cold water and soak for several hours or over night. In the morning, strain off the liquid and refrigerate. Each cup of the infusion can be gently warmed on the stove top before drinking.

Decoction: Add 1 1/2 teaspoons of slightly crushed fenugreek seeds and one teaspoon of anise to one cup of water and gently simmer on the stove top for 10 minutes. Drink three times per day.

Fenugreek Combinations:

Fenugreek can be taken in conjunction with alfalfa leaf, blessed thistle, marshmallow root, and red clover.

While you can combine one or more of these herbs, it is important to remember that specific combinations will work differently for every woman, so choose a combination that is best for you, and gauge your reaction and response to the combined supplements carefully. Divide the combined lactogenic treatment into three daily doses, taking each one before meals.

The recommended combination dosage is:

Fenugreek: Up to three capsules

Alfalfa leaf: Up to three capsules

Blessed thistle: Up to three capsules

Marshmallow Root: Up to three capsules

Red Clover: Up to 3 capsules

5. Goat's Rue

(Galega officinalis)

Also known as Holy Hay and French lilac, goat's rue, whose scientific name drives from gala (meaning milk) and ago (meaning "to bring on"), has become one of the most powerful and popular choices, alongside its sister herb fenugreek, as a potent galactogogue. Once native to the Middle East, this hardy perennial plant, which blooms particularly well in the summer months, has now been naturalized in Europe, western Asia, and western Pakistan, and extensively cultivated as a forage crop, an ornamental, and a bee plant. Goat's rue can also be found in Argentina, Chile, Ecuador, and New Zealand. In the early 1890s, it was introduced to the United States, in Utah, as a forage crop, and before the 1930s, was often collected in the states of Colorado, Connecticut, and New York, and before the population of goat's rue died out, it was a popular forage plant in the states of Maine and

Pennsylvania in the 1960s. Since the Middle Ages, goat's rue has been known for its ability to relieving the symptoms of diabetes, but until a less toxic alkaloid compound drawn from the plant was discovered in the 1920s, goat's rue was generally thought to be far too dangerous for human consumption because of its high toxicity levels. Although goat's rue is considered somewhat controversial, it remains a popular lactogenic herb for many women , and because very few problems associated with the consumption of this galactagogue have been reported, experienced herbalists are typically quite comfortable with recommending it as a supplement.

Goat's rue seems to be particularly beneficial to women who experience insufficient glandular tissue of the breast.

Non-Lactogenic Uses:

When combined with the use of other herbs, goat's rue can be used to stimulate the adrenal glands and pancreas, and is also used to treat diabetes, digestive problems, and as a diuretic, and blood purifier.

Warnings:

When using this herb, do not confuse it with rue. Fresh goat's rue is considered toxic. Dried goat's rue is considered safe for use in tinctures or teas. People currently being treated for diabetes should only use goat's rue under a doctor's supervision.

Allergies:

People who are allergic to soybeans, peanuts, legume, or green peas may also experience allergic reactions to goat's rue.

Pregnancy Information:

While mild amounts of goat's rue are thought to be relatively safe for most pregnant women, it is better to consult a qualified health care professional before taking this herb if you are currently pregnant.

Health Precautions:

Goat's rue might slow blood clotting and increase the risk of bleeding or bruising in people who suffer from blood disorders, so use with caution.

Medication Interactions:

Goat's rue may negatively affect certain medications used in the treatment of diabetes, such as glimepiride (Amaryl), glyburide (DiaBeta, Glynase PresTab, Micronase), insulin, pioglitazone (Actos), rosiglitazone (Avandia), chlorpropamide (Diabinese), glipizide (Glucotrol), and tolbutamide (Orinase).

Recommended Dosage as a Galactogogue:

As a tea: Pour one cup of boiling water over one teaspoon of dried goat's rue. Steep for five to 10 minutes. Sweeten to taste. Drink two to three cups of tea per day.

Tincture: Take one to two milliliters of tincture, or 10 to 15 drops beneath the tongue two to three times per day.

Chapter 2

Tinctures and Teas

When it comes to herbal supplements, some women prefer to take them as a liquid, in the form of a tincture or tea rather than as tablets or capsules, and this is a perfectly acceptable method of adding herbal supplements into your daily inducing routine.

Tinctures are liquid extracts made from herbs that you take orally. Although they are usually extracted in alcohol, which aids the herbs in releasing their medicinal properties while giving the tincture an indefinite shelf-life, they can also be extracted in vegetable glycerine or apple cider vinegar. Tinctures are easy and convenient to use, and because they are taken directly under the tongue, they enter the bloodstream much more directly than by any other means. Although some herbs will have an immediate effect, others may take several weeks of continual use before results are seen.

Tincture and teas are made from the same combination of herbs; they are simply taken differently. While teas need to be brewed before use, tinctures do not, which makes them a quick and convenient alternative. A bottle of tincture can be carried in a pocket or purse, and taken on the go.

Tinctures are usually contained in glass dropper bottles, and the dosage is measured by a dropper-full, in which a recommended adult dose of tincture would be two droppers-full of tincture taken beneath the tongue. Tinctures can sometimes have an unpleasant taste, so if you need to dilute them, you can add the drops to a cup of water or juice, or flavor the tincture with lemon and honey, and still receive the same medicinal benefits. You can also add two droppers-full of tincture to eight ounces of hot water to enjoy a cup of instant herbal tea.

Depending on their ingredient, many tinctures can be taken in conjunction with other breast-milk boosting herbal supplements. Once you have taken the tincture, it is best to wait 15 minutes before eating and drinking to ensure the herbs' effectiveness.

You can purchase nursing tinctures from a variety of online herbalists, or, if you prefer, you can follow the recipe below and learn how to make your own. This homemade tincture is said to boost milk supply and produce richer, creamier, highly nutritious breast milk.

Nursing Tincture

Ingredients:

1/2 cup Goat's Rue

1/2 cup Red Raspberry Leaf

1/2 cup Blessed Thistle

1/2 cup Fenugreek

1/2 cup Marshmallow Root

1/4 cup Fennel

High-proof vodka

Filtered water

Directions:

Place the measured herbs in a clean glass quart jar, and add just enough filtered water to wet them. Fill the jar with vodka. After tightly covering the jar, shake it well, and place it in a cool, dark place for 2-6 weeks. Shake the jar every few days.

After 2 weeks, the tincture may be used, but to receive the full medicinal properties, it is recommended that you allow it to brew for a minimum of 4 weeks. After 6 weeks, the alcohol will have drawn all medicinal properties from the herbs.

After the tincture has steeped, strain the herbs out of it, and pour the liquid into clean glass dropper bottles. Store in a cool, dark place.

You can take 2 droppers-full of this tincture 2-3 times per day.

Traditional Medicinals has produced and marketed Mother's Milk Tea since 1974, and this timeless herbal supplement alternative has been used by many women over the past 42 years with great success. Each tea bag, which is steeped in 8 ounces of hot water prior to drinking, contains a blend of bitter fennel, anise, coriander, fenugreek, blessed thistle, spearmint leaf, West Indian lemongrass, lemon verbena leaf, and marshmallow root, and the taste is often described as "sweet-bitter black licorice". A lot of women suggest flavoring the tea with lemon and honey to improve its strong taste. It is recommended that nursing women drink three to five cups of Mother's Milk Tea per day to increase their breast milk supply.

Mother's Milk Tea is easy to purchase, either in retail stores or online, and is conveniently pre-packaged and economical, but if you prefer, you may blend and brew your own nursing tea by following one of the recipes below. To steep loose-leaf tea, you can either place a tea-ball of herbs in your water, or directly add herbs to boiling water, and then strain before drinking.

Homemade Mother's Milk Tea 1

Ingredients:

1/2 cup dried Raspberry Leaf

1/2 cup dried Nettle Leaf

1/4 cup Fenugreek seeds

1/4 cup Fennel seeds

1/4 cup Alfalfa leaf

1/4 cup dried Chamomile flowers

1/4 cup Dandelion leaf

Directions:

Mix herbs together and store in a tightly sealed glass jar, placing the container in a cool, dark place. The herbs will be ready for immediate use.

To brew one cup of tea, add 1 tablespoon of herbs to 2 cups of boiling water, and simmer on the stove for 10-15 minutes. Strain and serve.

To make a gallon of tea, add 1/2 cup of herb mix to one gallon of boiling water, and simmer on the stove for 10-15 minutes. Strain. Store tea in refrigerator.

Drink 3-5 cups of tea per day.

Homemade Mother's Milk Tea 2

Ingredients:

1/2 cup dried Nettle Leaf

1/2 cup dried Red Raspberry Leaf

1/4 cup dried Alfalfa Leaf

1/4 cup dried Dandelion Leaf

1/4 cup Fennel seed

1/4 cup dried Blessed Thistle

Directions:

Mix herbs together, and store in a tightly sealed glass quart jar, placed in a cool, dark place. The herbs will be ready for immediate use.

To prepare one cup of tea, add 1 tablespoon of herbs to 1 cup of boiling water, and allow to steep, covered, for 15 minutes. Strain and serve.

You can make larger quantities of this nursing tea by increasing the amount of herbs and water you use during preparation, and brew as directed above. Store excess tea in your refrigerator.

Drink 3-5 cups of tea pr day.

Chapter 3

25 Breast Milk Boosting Super Foods

If you want to increase your breast milk supply naturally, and ensure that you are producing the most nutritious liquid gold possible, there is no better way to do this than by following a healthy, clean green lifestyle. By eliminating processed foods and raw sugars and incorporating fruits and vegetables, lean protein, and brown rice into your diet, while ensuring that you stay well-hydrated by drinking plenty of cool, refreshing water, you will see a noticeable difference in the quantity and quality of your breast milk. Here is a list of fantastic foods to get you started along the path to making rich, creamy, sweet super-charged milk.

1. Oatmeal

It is so simple to prepare a bowl of

heart-healthy, slow-cooking, old-fashioned oats. They are a fantastic breast milk booster, and are super-delicious when prepared with 1/4 cup almond milk, 1 tablespoon of coconut oil, and your favorite fruit.

2. Salmon

Salmon is a terrific source of Essential Fatty Acids (EFA) and Omega-3, which increase lactation and produce highly nutritious breast milk. Salmon is delicious when grilled or broiled. It can be lightly brushed with olive oil and lemon juice and seasoned with garlic and fresh dill.

3. Spinach and Beet Leaves

Spinach and beet leaves contain iron, calcium, and folic acid as well as detoxifying agents to prevent illness and boost the immune system of anemic nursing women. Both can be used in soups or flat bread recipes, and spinach makes the wonderful base for a nutritious salad.

4. Carrots

Carrots are high in vitamin A, and like spinach, they contain lactation producing qualities, and a glass of carrot juice with breakfast may do wonders for your milk supply. Carrots can be enjoyed raw, steamed, pureed, or even enjoyed in soups, During the winter, you might enjoy a bowl of warm pureed carrots served with almond milk and honey.

5. Fennel seeds

Fennel seeds can be used as a seasoning, tossed in a salad, or eaten as a snack. They can also be boiled in a cup of milk for a quick lactation drink.

6. Fenugreek seeds:

Like fennel, these milk-boosting seeds can be used as a seasoning, tossed in a salad, or eaten as a snack. They can also be added to pancake batter for a morning milk pick-me-up.

7. Bottle Gourd

Although not commonly thought of as a "typical" vegetable, the bottle gourd is a water-based veggie that keeps nursing women well-hydrated. Fresh bottle gourds can be peeled, stewed, and mashed, and you can season it to taste either savory (with spices and herbs) or sweet (with almond milk, coconut oil, and honey.)

8. Basil Leaves

Basil leaves provide you with anti-oxidants and help to boost the immune system while aiding in lactation. They are a delicious way to season soups and stews. You can also steep a few of these leaves in a cup of water. Drink it first thing in the morning to experience the almost-magical effects!

9. Garlic

Not only does it add wonderful flavor to prepared dishes, garlic is one of the best breast milk boosting super foods available to nursing women. It is rich with lactation and health benefits, as it can aid in the prevention of all cancers. Stir-fried garlic is a terrific addition to vegetables, casseroles, stews, and lean protein meals.

10. Barley

Barley helps to keep nursing women well-hydrated, and can be used in homemade soups and stews. You can also boil barley, and drink the water as a way to hydrate and increase milk supply.

11. Chickpeas

Chickpeas are chock-full of protein, calcium, B-vitamins, and fiber, and make a delicious snack when seasoned with garlic and lemon juice. They can be boiled and cooled and served in a salad, or consider making a batch of homemade hummus to eat with pita.

12. Asparagus

This "must-have" food for nursing women is high in fiber and vitamins A and K, and promotes the balance of hormones essential to lactation. An alternative to serving this vegetable as a side dish with dinner is to prepare an asparagus cocktail by finely chopping it and boiling it in a pan of milk. Simply strain out the asparagus and drink the milk for fantastic results.

13. Brown Rice

While providing an energy boost, brown rice also helps normalize hormonal mood swings and offers hormone stimulants to boost lactation.

14. Cumin Seeds

While cumin seeds are an excellent breast-milk booster and fat burner, they should be used in moderation. Add a pinch of cumin powder to a glass of milk every other day to aid in lactation and digestion.

15. Black Sesame Seeds:

While an excellent source of calcium, and very delicious when added to a glass of milk, try to limit how often you use black sesame seeds.

16. Oils and Fats:

While these should be used in moderation, it is very important to incorporate fats and oils into your diet, as they promote healthy lactation. Choose heart healthy oils such as olive, coconut, rice bran, or almond butter.

17. Apricots

Apricots, either fresh or dried, are rich in calcium and fiber, and help to balance hormones. They are delicious in oatmeal.

18. Cow's Milk

Cow's milk is high in EFA, so try to drink 2 or 3 glasses a day.

19. Dill Leaves

Dill leaves are high in fiber and vitamin K. They can be added to plain, non-fat yogurt to make a healthy vegetable dip.

20. Flax Seed

When adding flax seed to recipes, it is best to use flax seed meal, which is easier to digest.

Both flax seed meal and oil provide the same milk-boosting properties as the seeds.

21. Poppy Seeds

It is very important to relax while nursing, which helps to aid in the let-down reflex, and poppy seeds can act as a sedative to soothe and calm you. They are delicious roasted and add a pop of flavor to lemon muffins, but should be used sparingly.

22. Water and Juices

Staying well-hydrated increases total milk volume you produce per each nursing session while perfectly replenishing your body. Drink a glass of water or juice prior to--and right after--nursing.

23. Almonds

Almonds are rich in vitamin E and Omega-3, and are an excellent way to naturally balance nursing hormones. You can add them to salads or oatmeal, or simply eat them as a snack. Almond milk is good for you, too!

24. Sweet Potato

Sweet potatoes are packed with potassium, and provide a fatigue-fighting carbohydrate while providing an excellent source of vitamin C and B-complex. Sweet potatoes are wonderful baked, or mashed, and can be seasoned with savory spices or sweetened with cinnamon and honey.

25. Papaya

Papaya is a natural sedative and can help you relax while nursing. Toss it in an Asian salad, or eat it as a healthy snack.

These delicious and healthy super foods provide the nursing woman with a veritable smorgasbord of meal options. Mix and match them in any combination, and you'll soon be making a fountain of nutritious liquid gold fit for a king!

Part IV

For the Health and Well Being
of the Adult Nursing Couple

Chapter 1

H2O and Breast Milk Supply

Water is essential in promoting health and longevity. It relieves fatigue, improves mood, treats headaches and migraines, helps in digestion, aids in weight loss, and flushes toxins from our bodies. It's no surprise that consuming the proper daily intake of water is very much like drinking a cup full of liquid miracle. Not only does water help to keep our bodies perfectly balanced, it does wonders for lactation. Water actually increases the volume of breast milk a woman produces per each nursing session.

It is very common for a woman to feel thirsty while she is nursing, particularly during the let-down reflex when the breasts receive the deep stimulation required to encourage milk flow. Producing milk for another person's consumption can deplete your body and cause dehydration, so it is especially important that you drink plenty of H2O, particularly if you have begun to produce. Do your best to drink an 8-ounce glass of water 15-20 minutes before a nursing session, and if possible, drink a 4-ounce glass after nursing to ensure that you remain healthy and well-hydrated.

Every woman's recommended daily water intake is different and determined by her weight. To calculate your recommended daily water intake, simply divide your weight by two. The remainder will be the amount of water you should consume in ounces every day. I know, it probably seems like a lot, doesn't it? It isn't. It's actually perfect for you.

It is important to note that it is possible to over-hydrate, and drinking more than the recommended daily amount of water won't help to increase milk supply. Consuming your perfect daily allowance of H_2O will be sufficient to support and sustain a healthy supply of nutritious breast milk.

Chapter 2

Coping with Jaw Fatigue and
Gaining Suckling Stamina

If a medical condition known as Temporomandibular Joint Disorder (sometimes referred to as TMD) sounds quite painful, you're correct. It is. The temporomandibular joint is actually a hinge that connects your jaw to the temporal bones of the skull, which are in front of each ear. This joint allow you to move your jaw up and down and side to side so you are able to talk, chew, and yawn.

Although at this point there is no known cause for TMD, although medical professionals believe that the disorder's symptoms, which may include, but are not limited to, pain or tenderness in the face, jaw, neck, or ear, swelling on the side of the face, and difficulty opening the mouth wide, arise from problems with the jaw or, specifically, the joint itself, due to injury, grinding or clenching the teeth, and even stress. Unfortunately, suckling can exacerbate the condition, and this makes it very difficult to fully enjoy the nursing experience. Nursing should never be painful--for either partner. Jaw fatigue and discomfort can be very discouraging, and often a hindrance to everything that is wonderful about the loving nursing relationship.

The art of suckling takes a lot of dedicated work. Drawing milk from the breast, or even suckling within a dry nursing relationship, requires a strong latch that forces the nursing partner to open his mouth rather wide to ensure that he is taking in as much of the breast as he possibly can. As he begins the rhythmic motion of suckling, the jaws may flex, sometimes quite rapidly, as he stimulates the areola and nipple to encourage the let-down reflex. This is done in a series of short, rapid pulls, what I often refer to as "pacifier sucks", that can last from 3-5 minutes before milk begins to flow. Once the milk has been released, the nursing partner will often remain on the breast for an additional 10-15 minutes, so you can understand why suckling can be quite taxing. I often feel that the process of drawing milk from the breast is just as much a labor of love as making that lovely milk can be.

Even without the diagnosis of TMD, jaw fatigue is often a common problem within the dedicated adult nursing relationship, and building suckling stamina can take time and concentrated effort. During an interview that I conducted with my friend Mrs. D, she and her husband, Mr. E, openly discussed the challenge of facing this concern within their own long-term ANR. When preparing to write this chapter, I turned to this wonderful couple once more to ask Mr. E if he could give a bit of insight on the subject, and this is what he generously shared with me:

"My fatigue was brought on by the new experience of suckling. There was no previous condition of TMD. My symptom was mainly a tired, overworked feeling in the joint of my jaw, and that was the only discomfort I felt after about five minutes into the suckling experience. Fortunately, it didn't lead to anything else, such as headaches, neck pain, or earaches, and once I stopped suckling, the tired feeling in my jaw subsided.

"As far as remedies go for working through this? Practice, practice, practice! Seriously, just experiment with different positions. We came to the realization that I was more comfortable nursing in any position that allowed Mrs. D's breast to fall naturally into my mouth as oppose to positions that forced me to do more work by pulling in or suckling upward. One device we did come across is a half-moon nursing pillow by JJ Cole that we use for alternate positions, and it helps a lot. Since we've made position adjustments and began to consistently nurse, I haven't had any further issues.

"I would say that I have grown accustomed to the art of suckling. I don't think it is something that anyone could automatically know how to do from the start. I think what someone is trying to accomplish, and the motivation and determination behind it, is going to play into how long it will take to improve stamina. I'm quite sure it will happen sooner for some than others. It truly depends on the couple."

Proper suckling actually requires a concentrated focus on the lips and the muscles of the mouth rather than on the jaw. Once they have created a seal around the breast, the lips move continuously along the areola, flexing in an up and down motion that provides excellent stimulation and allows the breast to move freely in the mouth. When properly suckling, the chin will be tucked slightly beneath the breast, and this helps to prevent nursing fatigue.

You might find it helpful to nurse in sets. To do this, suckle just until you begin to feel the onset of jaw fatigue, and then rest until your jaw feels relaxed once more, before you proceed with suckling. You can repeat this process throughout the length of the suckling session. (Suckle for five minutes, rest for five, and repeat.)

To prepare the jaw for the impending suckling experience, it can often be beneficial to begin with a short series of jaw stretching exercise to loosen and relax the temporomandibular joint. They're very simple to do, and quite effective. Just open your mouth as widely as you possibly can, as if you're yawning, and then slowly bring the lower jaw upward without allowing the upper and lower teeth to meet. Afterwards, apply a warm, moist towel to the jaw for 3-5 minutes to sustain the loose and relaxed feeling of the joint.

To ease post-nursing discomfort, you can take an over-the-counter anti-inflammatory medication, such as ibuprofen, to help with muscle pain; if you're unable to take ibuprofen, acetaminophen may also help. Cool compresses or moist heat applied to the jaw are also helpful, and remember to relax! Stay focused while suckling, but don't concentrate so hard that you begin to tense up and clench the jaw. Keep your jaw loose and relaxed to ensure a beautiful and pain-free nursing experience!

While theses are just a few tips and tricks offered to you by long-term nursers, remember that you can always visit your health care provider if the problem persists, or you feel that you may be suffering from TMD. He or she will be able to provide proper treatment for your condition.

Practice really does make perfect. Over time, as you grow accustomed to the art of suckling, your stamina will improve, and the technique will become second nature to you!

Chapter 3

The Importance of Knowing your Breasts

How many times have we seen our breasts? They are two very beautiful things that evoke our femininity, and are am undeniably large part of our womanhood. We are familiar with their shape and size, the unique colorations and forms of the nipples and areolae, and while every breast is lovely, and a blessing to behold, how well do we know them? Can we recognize obvious changes? Do we fully understand what our normal is? Breast health is so important, and it's often easy to overlook; change is frightening–even when some transformations are perfectly natural, due to genetics, age, weight loss (or gain), menses, and pregnancy and/or lactation, but it's very important to know your body and define the world "normal".

When it comes to breasts–and particularly the nipples–normal is defined as the breasts you are born with. Nipples are often classified in three very specific ways: 1. Everted, 2. Inverted, and 3. Retracted. Inverted or retracted nipples are not always a sign of a worrisome breast condition or serious illness; if you were born with either of these conditions, then this is your normal. However, nipple change should always be discussed with a qualified healthcare professional to be certain that an underlying problem is not present.

When lactation begins to occur, there will be physical changes in your breasts. They may swell and ache; you may experience tenderness at the outer sides (where the first size increase typically occurs) and in your underarms. The body of the breast may hold small warm spots; you might even experience little shooting twinges of growing pains–or notice tiny lumps and bumps that have never been present before.

The areolae often increase in diameter and darken in color, and the nipples sometimes widen and change shape. You might even notice tiny prominent "bumps" popping up along the surface of your areolae–these are Montgomery glands, and are a perfectly natural occurrence in beautiful brand new nursing breasts.

All of these changes are normal, and should be celebrated as you begin the lovely journey into lactation.

Once you have established lactation, and your body has grown accustomed to the milk-making process, you will begin to recognize your new "normal", which is probably much different than the "normal" you once knew to be your breasts, and any changes that vary from what you know.

And, chances are, your partner will

recognize them, too.

I think it is very important for a man to know this "normal". Allow him to learn every inch of your breasts through sight and touch.

Mr. S often gives me breast massages–and has even assisted me with breast self-exams to ensure that what he and I both recognize as my normal remains that way. It is an intimate–and very soothing–way to practice proper breast health care at home.

Always take care of your precious ta-tas! And, remember, no matter how you define your normal, they are not merely practical, but pretty and perfect–and made just as unique as you!

Chapter 4

Nursing with Inverted Nipples

Nipples come in all shapes and sizes, and while most protrude, making the nursing experience a relatively carefree one, there are variations to size and shape that can make nursing difficult--but not impossible.

During suckling, the nursing partner stretches a woman's nipple forward and presses it upward against the roof of his mouth, but because he suckles at breast tissue rather than on the nipple, nursing should be feasible even if your nipples are inverted, as a strong latch and vigorous suckling will often draw them forward.

Some nipples are flat rather than inverted, and you can perform a pinch test to determine whether yours are flat or truly inverted. Grasp your breast at the edge of the areola between your thumb and index finger, and press in firmly, about one inch behind the nipple. If it does not protrude or become erect, it is flat, and if it retracts or disappears entirely, it is inverted. Severely inverted nipples will not respond to stimulation or cold by becoming erect.

An inverted nipple is caused by adhesions at the base of the nipple that bind the skin to the underlying tissue. As you approach full lactation, the breast skin does stretch a bit, but some of the cells in the nipple and areola may remain attached. Vigorous suckling can cause the adhesions to lift rather than breaking them loose, which can make the nursing experience painful and unpleasant.

Breasts function independently of one another, which is why it is not uncommon that a woman may have only one flat or inverted nipple. Degrees of inversion vary greatly; some inverted nipples can be pulled out manually while others disappear entirely during compressions. How difficult nursing will be is determined on the severity of the inversion--and on your partner's ability to properly suckle.

The Hoffman Technique is a simple manual exercise that can be used to break the adhesions of an inverted nipple. Place the thumbs of both hands opposite one another at the base of the nipple, and then gently, but firmly, pull the thumbs away from one another, both in an up and down and sideways motion. Begin by performing the Hoffman Technique twice a day, working up to five times per day.

Using a breast pump directly before nursing is also a wonderful way to draw the nipple out. Breast pumps can aid in breaking the adhesions that bind an inverted nipple by applying uniform pressure at the center of the nipple. If your partner opens his mouth widely enough, closing his lips firmly around the areola and pulling inward with a bit of vigorous force, he may easily be able to draw an inverted nipple forward, and over time, the nipple may respond to vigorous suckling and pose no further issues.

Do your best to avoid engorgement. Aside from being extremely painful, this condition can cause nipple to flatten against the areola, which can pose an even bigger nursing challenge if you naturally have flat or inverted nipples.

Unless your nipple retracts, you can stimulate it by grasping it and rolling it between your thumb and index finger for 30 seconds; after this form of manual stimulation, touch it with a cold, moist cloth, and then put your partner immediately to the breast.

Offering the breast is done differently by women with flat or inverted nipples than for those with protruding nipples. In this case, you should pull back on the areola to aid in the proper latch. Cup your breast in one hand, thumb placed on top with your fingers resting beneath it, and pull back on the breast, drawing it into the chest wall, which may help your nipple to protrude.

Some degree of nursing soreness is common for women with inverted nipples. After suckling, if the nipple retracts once more, this can cause moisture to become trapped, so gently pat the breast dry after every session. If the nipple is not drawn out during suckling and remains buried in breast tissue, your partner may be compressing it while nursing. You can apply a lanolin cream to soothe nursing discomfort.

In most cases, only one nipple is inverted, so you and your partner can certainly enjoy the nursing experience by suckling on the opposite breast as you pump to loosen the adhesions on the inverted nipple. Sometimes, a nipple can be drawn out after just one effective pumping sessions, while other women find that it takes a much longer period of time. It is wonderful to know, however, that generally, regardless of how long it may take, adhesion can always be loosened or broken to ensure successful nursing. While suckling on the inverted nipple, your partner may find that it retracts during the session. If you choose to do so, you can detach him from the breast to pump until the nipple is drawn forward once more, before putting him back on the breast. This takes time and patience, of course, but the end result of your laborious effort can be very rewarding.

Always remember, your partner is not nipple feeding. He is breastfeeding; once he successfully draws the nipple out, its shape really doesn't matter much at all.

Chapter 5

Breast Engorgement

Engorgement presents itself as a very real possibility to every lactating woman. This painful condition occurs when a woman's breasts become overfull with milk. The breast and areola may feel hard, swollen, and warm, and the skin may stretch and appear shiny. You may experience tenderness in the breast and underarm area, or run a low-grade fever, and the nipple may expand in diameter and lie flat against the areola, making latching quite difficult and nursing quite painful. The condition can occur in the areola and body of either one or both breasts, build to a peak before decreasing, remain at the same level for an extended period of time, or even peak several times. The best way to alleviate engorgement is to remove the surplus of milk from your breasts.

If possible, allow your partner to nurse, as suckling properly empties the breast; if he finds that he is having trouble latching, you should try to hand express your breast(s) prior to nursing. The release relieves nipple tension, making it easier for your partner to latch. Engorged breasts are often stubborn breasts, and may be slow in releasing milk. If your partner finds that after five minutes of oral massage, that he is unable to coax milk from the breast, ask him to nurse from the opposite side for several minutes before returning to the first breast. Repeatedly switching sides is sometimes beneficial. If he has remained on the stubborn breast for 20 minutes without results, remove him from the breast. You can then apply massage techniques, gentle breast compressions, or hand expression in an attempt to shift your milk. Warm compresses can be applied to the breast, too, or you might enjoy a soothing soak in the tub, or relaxing under a shower spray. Just be sure not to overheat, as this can make engorgement worse. Afterwards, if you are comfortable doing so, you can allow your partner to nurse once more. Sometimes, the breast will suddenly "give", releasing milk in solid form that then allows the flow to occur more naturally. These milk solids, while unexpected and a bit painful to release, are safe for your partner to consume.

Hand expression is often a better choice than a breast pump when it comes to relieving engorgement. Over-pumping to repeatedly empty the breasts in rapid succession to ease discomfort, can actually cause the breasts to fill more quickly, making the condition worse. It is best to gradually hand express milk, just a little at a time, to alleviate pressure and pain while emptying the breasts.

Cool compresses used in 20-minute intervals help to ease the discomfort for many women. Be sure to place a cloth between the ice pack and your breast to protect the skin. Avoid excess stimulation of the affected breast; for example, do not allow the shower to spray directly on the breast, avoid extended heat and pumping sessions, and do not restrict your fluid intake. Stay well-hydrated, as limiting fluids will not aid in eliminating engorgement.

Reverse Pressure Softening (RPS) is a technique that can be used in women suffering from moderate to severe engorgement to soften the areola to allow for easier latching. The method involves applying positive pressure to a 1-2 inch area of the areola, at the base of the nipple, to temporarily move some swelling upward and backward into the breast. RPS is safe and effective, and can be used as often as necessary.

To employ this technique, you may use either one or both hands, and any combination of fingers. Using the one hand method, begin by placing your fingers on the areola, directly at the base of the nipple, and curl your fingers inward, toward the chest, applying firm pressure that you will hold for a minimum of 60 seconds. In this form of Reverse Pressure Softening, the palm of the hand will rest against the breast, and the fingers will be pointing downward, with the nipple positioned between two spread fingers just below the first knuckle of each. The fingertip then curl into the areola at the base of the nipple. Repeat this process in sections along the areola, sliding your fingers so they overlap the previously treated area. RPS can take as long as 10-20 minutes to perform, and you shouldn't be surprised if it causes temporary dimpling or pitting of the areola. Applied pressure should be firm, but never painful. To ease discomfort, simply use less pressure, and apply the technique for longer periods of time. The length of the RPS session will depend on your level of engorgement.

Your partner can help you with RPS, too. It is often beneficial if he performs the technique from behind, by sliding his hands over your shoulders, and then employing the same finger placement and motions that you would use during the one hand RPS method.

For generations, cabbage leaves have been used as an effective form of engorgement relief. Simply separate and wash a head of green cabbage, and blot dry. Apply the leaves to engorged breasts for up to 20 minutes three times a day. The leaves can be chilled or used at room temperature, but you should not use them for more than the recommended length of time, as cabbage is known to impede milk supply.

For further relief of engorgement pain, you can make a simple fenugreek poultice by boiling several ounces of fenugreek seeds in a small amount of water. Transfer the boiled seeds into a bowl and mash them. You can then apply the mashed seeds to your breasts and cover them with a thin cloth.

Engorgement will often clear in time, but if the problem persists, or you find that your breasts are not responsive to these treatment methods, it is recommended that you consult a lactation consultant or medical professional for advice and proper treatment.

Chapter 6

Plugged Milk Ducts

A plugged, or blocked, milk duct is an area of the breast where milk flow is obstructed, and the problem is often caused by engorgement or inadequate milk removal, infrequent or skipped nursings or other expression sessions, pressure on the duct, inflammation due to injury, a bacterial or yeast infection, or an allergy. Stress, fatigue, anemia, or a weakened immune system can also cause obstructions. The nipple pore may be blocked, or the obstruction may occur further up in the ductal system. This condition normally occurs gradually, and is commonly seen in only one breast. A plugged milk duct will often cause a hard lump or wedge-shaped area in the breast that is red, hot, swollen, and painful. A plug may often shift, and, typically, the pain is more severe prior to nursing, and during the let-down reflex, and lessens after milk is emptied from the breast. Women sometimes run a light fever of 101.3 when suffering this condition.

When a milk duct is blocked, you may notice a decrease in your milk output, but with frequent nursings and pumping sessions, this problem will normally be remedied once your condition improves. During expression, your breast milk may be stringy, grainy, or quite thick, and once the blockage is cleared, it is not uncommon to experience a tender or bruised feeling in the affected breast for a week or more afterward. It is important that you do not stop nursing, as this can lead to an abscess in the breast. Below are some things you can do if you believe you are suffering from plugged milk ducts.

Supportive Measures:

Get plenty of rest

Drink plenty of fluids

Eat nutritious foods to aid your immune system

Nursing Management:

Nurse or express often, making sure to thoroughly empty your breasts

Before nursing, apply a warm compress and gently massage the breast

Loosen your bra and wear non-restrictive clothing to aid in milk flow

Nurse on the affected side first. If this becomes too painful, switch to the opposite breast after the let-down reflex has occurred

Apply gentle breast massage or compressions while nursing

After nursing, hand express, and then apply cool compresses to the breast

Antibiotics are normally not prescribed to treat blocked milk ducts. You can ease inflammation and discomfort by taking ibuprofen, or if you are unable to take ibuprofen for any reason, acetaminophen may help.

Chapter 7

Mastitis

Mastitis is an inflammation of the breast that is normally caused by milk stasis, an obstruction of milk flow, rather than an infection. While mastitis can become very serious and lead to an abscess of the breast, non-infectious mastitis (more common) that lasts for less than 24 hours can often be treated with milk removal and at-home supportive care. If the condition worsens, or affects both breasts, antibiotics should be started immediately. Mastitis can be caused by blocked milk ducts, or from an infection that has entered the body through a particular entry point, normally cracked or bleeding nipples. The condition normally affects only one breast, and comes on quite sudden;y. Stress, fatigue, infrequent or skipped nursings and expressions, inadequate milk removal, anemia, or a weakened immune system can also lead to this painful condition.

Mastitis symptoms are similar to those of plugged milk ducts (swollen, tender, hot, and reddened breasts), but much more severe; red streaks will often appear around the affected area. Mastitis can cause a woman to run a fever of 101.3 degrees or higher, and she may experience chills, body aches, and other flu-like symptoms. During expression, breast milk may be lumpy, clumpy, gelatinous, or stringy, or contain mucus, pus, or blood. Despite its appearance, the milk will still be safe for consumption, although its flavor may be much saltier, due to iron and chloride content.

If you believe you have mastitis, you should start treatment immediately. The following at-home care treatments may help you with this.

Supportive Measures:

Get plenty of bed rest

Increase your fluid intake

Nursing Management:

Nurse or express often, making sure to thoroughly empty your breasts

Before nursing, apply a warm compress and gently massage the breast

Loosen your bra and wear non-restrictive clothing to aid in milk flow

Nurse on the affected side first. If this becomes too painful, switch to the opposite breast after the let-down reflex has occurred

Apply gentle breast massage or compressions while nursing

After nursing, hand express, and then apply cool compresses to the breast

Although it is perfectly acceptable (and recommended) for you to nurse from the affected breast, your partner may not be comfortable doing this; it is vital that milk is removed completely from the breast, so be certain to pump and/or hand express often. If, after following these supportive nursing measures, you are still symptomatic, be sure to see your doctor right away.

Chapter 8

Milk Blisters

A milk blister, or bleb, is a blocked nipple pore that occurs when a tiny bit of skin overgrows a milk duct opening and milk backs up behind it. A milk blister is often a small, painful white, clear, or yellow dot on the nipple or areola, and the pain is focused on that spot or directly behind it. During breast compressions when milk is forced down the duct, a bleb will typically bulge outward. Milk blisters can be persistent and very painful during nursing, and may last for several days, or even weeks, before spontaneously disappearing when the skin peels away from them. These blisters differ from friction blisters, which often appear as red or brown spots on the nipple, and are caused by an improper latch or ill-fitting breast pump flange or nipple shield.

To treat milk blisters, it is often helpful to apply moist heat to the breast prior to nursing, as this tends to soften the blister, and several times a day, before applying the moist heat, you can incorporate a saline soak to aid in opening the pores and promote healing. Dissolve 2 teaspoons of Epsom salt in a small amount of hot water, and then add enough cool water to make 1 cup of solution. After soaking in the solution, place a hot, moist towel to the blister, or use a cotton ball soaked in olive oil to soften the bleb. You may saline soak four times per day.

While nursing or pumping may often help the skin to expand so the bleb will open on its own, you can clear the skin away from it by rubbing the blister with a moist washcloth. If a plug appears from the nipple, you can use clean fingers to pull it from the pore. The bleb can also be opened with the use of a sterile needle, but this procedure should only be done by a health care professional, as the risk of infection is very high if you attempt this on your own.

Nurse or pump on the affected side first if possible, and be sure to treat the milk blister after every expression session.

Chapter 9

Breast Care for the Nursing Woman

Proper breast care is important for every woman, but it plays a key role in the nursing woman's life, as healthy, well-cared for breasts can help to prevent medical conditions, such as infections and thrush.

Tender or sore nipples are very common in new-to-nursing women, and are usually caused by a poor or improper latch. Always check your partner's position, and ensure that he is employing the proper latch technique. There are many lanolin-based over the counter non-prescription nursing creams available, and these are wonderful to help dull and soothe nursing discomfort. A small amount can be applied to the nipples prior to nursing, and because they are non-toxic and safe for human consumption, they will not need to be washed off before your partner comes to the breast. Cool compresses may also help to dull nursing pain, or you might consider purchasing gel nursing pads, which can be stored in the refrigerator, and then tucked into your bra to provide soothing relief.

Dry or itchy nipples are also common within the first weeks. Coconut oil is very helpful when massaged onto the breasts, and some women use vinegar to cure itchy nipples. To do this, mix 1 tablespoon of white vinegar into a cup of water, saturate a cotton ball with the solution, and place it over the affected area for 3-5 minutes. Afterwards, lean over a sink and slowly pour the remaining vinegar and water mixture over your nipples.

Itchy nipples can be a sign of a more serious medical condition known as thrush, or nipple thrush. Thrush is a fungal infection that often enters the breast through a damaged nipple, and should be treated properly by a medical professional.

Thrush can occur in one or both breasts, and the pain, which is often described as a burning, itching, or stinging sensation in the nipples, can radiate through the body of the breast as sharp shooting jabs or a deep, dull ache, and is worse just after nursing and in between expressions. The nipple may become bright pink and the areola may redden or become dry and flaky; sometimes, a fine white rash will appear on the breast. Thrush is contagious and can be transferred to your partner; if this happens, you will both need to be treated for the condition.

Wash your breasts thoroughly after each nursing session, using a mild anti-bacterial soap, and be sure to rinse them completely with warm water. Dry your breasts carefully to prevent moisture from forming and dust the undersides with a light sprinkling of cornstarch. Change your nursing pads frequently.

If you notice breaking skin or damage to the nipple (cracks, fissures, or bleeding), be sure to remedy the problem right away, as these are common entry points for serious infections. You can care for your nipples by following the above suggestions, and then applying an over the counter anti-bacterial ointment such a Neosporin, or even Carmex lip therapy. Surprisingly, this works very well to aid in healing! If you are already producing, you can apply breast milk to affected nipples, and allow it to dry. Breast milk contains fabulous natural healing properties.

By caring for your breasts, you'll be sure to enjoy a pleasant--and healthy-- nursing experience!

Chapter 10

Discussing Lactation with your Doctor

All women who induce non-maternal lactation or choose to re-lactate will eventually face the issue of discussing this with their health care provider. It can be difficult and even embarrassing to broach such a sensitive subject, but it truly is important that you do.

Lactation brings many changes to the female breast, and these changes can often mimic very serious medical conditions, including cancer. During an examination, your doctor may notice these change, and order further testing. All breast changes show up in mammograms that can be read inaccurately if the issue is not addressed.

The best way to tell your doctor about your lactation journey is during a scheduled appointment or routine examination. Be open and honest. There should be no reason that you will need to explain why you have chosen to induce lactation, so, if you're uncomfortable sharing the specifics of your ANR with others, this should not be a problem; simply let him or her know that you have elected to lactate, and explain that you felt s/he should know prior to your check-up.

If your doctor is curious about your decision, and some may be, you can openly discuss your reasons for lactation, whether they be for physical pain relief, nutritional aspects, or simply for the pure joy of the experience. Doctors are professionals; they have seen and heard many things throughout the length of their careers, so induced lactation should come as no surprise (or shock) to them.

No matter how you choose to discuss lactation with your doctor, always remember that honesty is the best policy, and can prevent the need for further unnecessary testing, which is stressful and expensive.

Chapter 11

Routine Mammograms and Lactation

Every woman understands the importance of having routine mammograms to ensure the health of her beautiful breasts, but there is sometimes the question as to whether a woman can--or should--have a mammogram if she is lactating. The answer to this is quite simple: A lactating woman can have a mammogram; as a matter of fact, it is during this time that an annual mammogram becomes even more important because lactation can make small lumps harder to detect during routine breast self-exams.

Because lactating breasts can make it more difficult to read the mammogram's results, as milk production causes the breast tissue to become denser, it's recommended that women nurse just before their mammograms to empty their breasts, or even request a radiologist who specializes in reading the x-rays of lactating women.

Due to increased tenderness and sensitivity, mammograms may be slightly more painful for nursing women, but the x-rays are perfectly safe and do not harm the quality of breast milk.

So, not only is it perfectly fine to have a mammogram during lactation, it is highly recommended. You should definitely keep your scheduled mammograms, even while enjoying a healthy ANR!

Chapter 12

Proper Breast Milk Handling and Storage

Breast milk is one of the healthiest foods a person will ever consume. As a matter of fact, it is so vitamin and nutrient-enriched that medical research now shows that this "liquid gold" is just as beneficial for adults as it is for infants, and research has concluded that an adult can actually thrive, not merely survive, on a diet consisting of only breast milk.

Remember, this is the good stuff, the pure stuff, and it is unadulterated with artificial additive and preservatives, so to truly reap all of the fantastic health benefits that breast milk naturally provides, it needs to be handled and stored properly. Here's how you can do this!

Preparing to Store Fresh Breast Milk:

•Prior to expressing, be sure to wash your hands to prevent transferring bacteria to your breast milk. You should actually do this before nursing, too, and be sure that your breasts are free of lotions, perfumes, and powders.

•Store collected milk in either screw-cap bottles, hard plastic cups with tight-fitting lids, or breast milk storage bags, which are sterile, BPA free, freezer-safe, and designed specifically for proper milk storage. It isn't recommended that breast milk is stored in traditional freezer bags or other plastic bags.

•Be sure to label your containers with the date of expression, and use the oldest breast milk first.

•You shouldn't mix "old" and "new" breast milk together in one container.

•I know...I know...breast milk is a precious commodity, and you don't want to waste a drop, but be sure to discard any unused and left-over milk. No hoarding!

•Breast milk bags are disposable, and should be thrown away after each use.

•Wash your breast pump after each use.

How to Thaw Frozen Breast Milk:

•The best (and safest) way to thaw frozen breast milk is by transferring it from the freezer to the refrigerator, but if you need it in a hurry, you can thaw your milk more quickly by swirling the storage container in a bowl of warm water. Breast milk will often separate, and you may notice that the "cream" has risen to the top. This is perfectly normal, and the milk is safe for drinking. Swirling the container (either in a bowl of warm water as it thaws or after thawing) will usually help to mix the separated layers of milk.

•Don't thaw frozen breast milk in a microwave oven.

•Once thawed, breast milk should never be re-frozen. (I know...there's that waste not, want not thing again...)

Storage Methods and Duration of Fresh Breast Milk:

If you're planning to use your breast milk fairly soon after expression, it can be left out at room temperature, up to 77 degrees F or 25 degrees C, for 6-8 hours. To preserve its freshness, you can cover the collection container with a cool, dry towel.

Insulated Cooler Bag: A cooler comes in very handy while traveling, or if you're planning a vacation. The bag's internal temperature should remain between 5 and 39 degrees F or -15 and 4 degrees C. Keep ice packs in contact with your breast milk at all times, and be sure to limit how often you open the cooler bag. If using this method of storage, milk will stay fresh for 24 hours.

Refrigerator: With a temperature of 39 degrees F or 4 degrees C, breast milk can be safely stored in this way for up to 5 days. Try to place your milk in the back of the fridge where it is cooler if possible.

Freezer Compartment of a Refrigerator: As long as the temperature remains at 5 degrees F or -15 degrees C, breast milk can be stored safely here for 2 weeks.

Freezer Compartment of a Refrigerator with Separate Doors: If you choose to freeze your breast milk, a freezer with an internal temperature of 0 degrees F or -18 degrees C will preserve the milk's freshness for 3-6 months.

Chest or Upright Deep Freezer: If you choose to freeze your milk in this way, at a temperature of -4 degrees F or -20 degrees C, it will remain fresh and perfectly safe for drinking for 6-12 months.

To further ensure the quality of your breast milk, store your containers at the back of the freezer if you can; the temperature is much more consistent, and this preserves all of those fantastic lipids in your milk!

Remember, contrary to what others may think, breast milk is a food, not a human waste, so preserve yours carefully for future use. Consider using it in recipes, substituting cow's milk with your milk, as a health or beauty remedy, or even donating it to bless others! When it comes to the use of fresh and healthy breast milk, the possibilities are endless!

AFTERWORD

AND

ACKNOWLEDGEMENTS

Well, dear reader, we have finally reached the conclusion of *The Art of Lactation*, and while this book has come to an end, your personal journey into the beautiful world of lactation has truly just begun. I certainly hope this guidebook will continue to be a great help to you as you pursue the beauty of this magnificent process in your own life.

I wish you great success, much happiness, and smooth travels along the way, and May the journey be a blessing in your life.

In closing, I would like to take a minute to thank a group of very special ladies who were on hand to answer questions and provide timely and accurate information throughout the writing of this book: registered nurse Holly

S., board certified lactation consultants, Christy K. and Rebecca D., and certified herbalist Elaine R. Your generosity in sharing your knowledge, as well as your support and encouragement, is such a blessing in my life.

Thank you to Mr. E for contributing so generously to this book, and to both he and his lovely wife, Mrs. D, for being such kind supporters of the ANR community. Meeting you has been a true pleasure.

And, of course, without Mr. S' unfailing support and faith in me, I could never have achieved all that I have--or become the woman I am.

Warmly,

The Loving Milk Maid

ABOUT THE AUTHOR

Known to readers around the world as The Loving Milk Maid (or simply LMM), freelance writer and blogger Jennifer Elisabeth Maiden gained recognition with the launch of her original blog, Bountiful Fruits: A Loving ANR Journey, and now runs the successful website Bountiful Fruits, which explores the fascinating world of the adult nursing relationship and provides visitors with information on lactation, breastfeeding, relationships, intimacy, sex, and marriage, and the podcast Bountiful Fruits ANR Chat with the Loving Milk Maid. The Loving Milk Maid is an ANR/ABR advocate and educator who believes in promoting positive body image, recognition of the beautiful female anatomy, and happily-ever-afters, and is the author of several books, including *The Art of Lactation* and *A Garden of Gold*. She and her husband, Mr. S, reside in Ohio where she is currently working on her fifth   book, *Bountiful Blessings: Living the Adult Nursing Lifestyle in Everyday Life.*

Made in United States
Orlando, FL
20 April 2024

46009514R00147